The Orange Book
Of
Athletic Training
Certification Exam
Practice Questions

———

5 Full-Length Practice Exams

Chad Dufrene, MA, ATC, LAT

This publication is designed to provide accurate and authoritative information in regard to the subject matter covered. It is sold with the understanding that neither the author nor the publisher is engaged in rendering legal, investment, accounting or other professional services. While the publisher and author have used their best efforts in preparing this book, they make no representations or warranties with respect to the accuracy or completeness of the contents of this book and specifically disclaim any implied warranties of merchantability or fitness for a particular purpose. No warranty may be created or extended by sales representatives or written sales materials. The advice and strategies contained herein may not be suitable for your situation. You should consult with a professional when appropriate. Neither the publisher nor the author shall be liable for any loss of profit or any other commercial damages, including but not limited to special, incidental, consequential, personal, or other damages.

Book Cover by Chad Dufrene using www.canva.com

Illustrations by Chad Dufrene using www.canva.com

The Board of Certification, Inc. (BOC) Examination is created, owned, and managed by the Board of Certification, Inc. At no point in this publication's creation was specific BOC Examination content from the past and present used. The 5 Domains referenced in this publication are property of the Board of Certification, Inc. Permission to reference the Domains are strictly reserved by the Board of Certification, Inc.

Edited by Alyssa Dufrene

First edition 2024

Disclaimers

The purpose of this publication is to provide practice for the Board of Certification Examination. It is not intended to serve as a comprehensive study aid. It is strongly recommended that you refer to the guidelines and instructions provided by the Board of Certification, Inc. for further information.

For information regarding this publication's reference materials, please refer to the section entitled "Bibliography."

The information provided in this book is not intended to be used to provide medical or legal advice.

The domains are not listed or explained in this book. Just the associated numbers are provided with the answers. For information regarding the domains, refer to the BOC website (bocatc.org).

Acknowledgments

I would like to start out by thanking my good friend and former colleague, Erin Kennedy, for her guidance and support through the process of writing this book. This book would also not be possible without the knowledge and guidance imparted through the years from Cary Berthelot, Karen Lew Feirman, Rhonda Cross Beemer, Edward Hebert, Bovorn Sirikul, Ralph Wood, Gary Lewis, Scott Arceneaux, Justin Fleetwood, Brett Cascio, Troy Bourgeois, Wame Waggenspack, Winston Riehl and Ray Castle.

I would like to thank the following friends and family members for their support: Brad Borland, Greg Reeves, Jason Rees, Arden Ballard, Lou and Eileen Dominguez, Larry Apken, Brian Dufrene, Fuller and Molly Lyon, and Jim and Sandra Lyon.

I dedicate this book in memory of my late parents, Floyd and Erna Bailey. I would also like to dedicate this book to my late athletic training profession mentors and friends, Robert Goodwin, Josh Yellen, and Bryan Sentilles.

Most of all, I would like to thank my "editor-in-chief" and better half, Alyssa, for being a model of inspiration, a mother, a best friend, a taskmaster, and now a marathoner. You and Adam are the two people in the world that I want to make the most proud of me.

Table of Contents

Introduction

The Board of Certification (BOC) took over credentialing of the Athletic Training profession 72 years after Dr. S.E. Bilik authored *The Trainer's Bible* in 1917. The BOC was charged with the Herculean task of producing an exam to test the requisite knowledge of an entry-level professional. That was in 1989 when the White House was inhabited by President Ronald Reagan. Tim Burton's Batman was tops in the box office, and the top song was "Look Away" by Chicago. The BOC Exam has evolved a lot since Michael Keaton donned fake muscles and launched Jack Nicholson's Joker off of a Gotham City highrise. However, it is still the same worthy adversary that thousands have faced over the years. In fact, it is an adversary so worthy that 628 of the 2,427 first-timers between 2022-2023 did not pass. I would venture to say that the most common question amongst those 628 test-takers was the same as all Athletic Training Program faculty and staff have had over the years: Why did students not pass the BOC? I could not find a definitive answer to that question during my 10-year tenure as an Athletic Training Program faculty member. However, I did find that there was a direct correlation between the amount of simulated exam practice and higher scores on the BOC, and this book provides just that. In fact there are 5 full-length practice exams in this book. Each practice exam contains a combination of multiple choice, choose all that apply multiple choice, matching, and hot-spot questions. You can utilize them at your leisure, but I would recommend using them under a simulated environment. The answer pages follow each exam, and they contain the BOC domains associated with each answer. I would like to congratulate you for getting this far and would like to wish you the best of luck in your preparation. I look forward to soon calling you a colleague.

Exam 1 on Next Page

1. The pronator teres of the forearm is innervated by which nerve?

    a. median nerve

    b. radial nerve

    c. ulnar nerve

    d. posterior interosseous nerve

    e. anterior interosseous nerve

2. _____refers to the formation of bone in places that it should not form in the body.

    a. Osteochondritis dissecans

    b. Osteosarcoma

    c. Myositis ossificans

    d. Osteomyelitis

    e. Paget's disease

3. _____is characterized as a fracture of the distal radius with dorsal displacement of the bone.

    a. Smith's fracture

    b. Colles' fracture

    c. Bennett's fracture

    d. Jones fracture

    e. Nightstick fracture

4. _____is the leading cause of sudden cardiac death among youth athletes.

    a. Hypertrophic cardiomyopathy

    b. Marfan syndrome

    c. Commotio cordis

    d. Aortic dissection

    e. Cardiac tamponade

5. During the_____phase of healing, one should begin strengthening and neuromuscular control exercises.

    a. inflammation

    b. proliferation

    c. remodeling

    d. maturation

    e. all of the above

6. During the_____technique of proprioceptive neuromuscular facilitation, the patient voluntarily moves the limb until resistance, holds against isometric resistance, and relaxes while the agonist contracts.

    a. contract-relax

    b. hold-relax

    c. slow-reversal-hold-relax

    d. hold-relax-hold

    e. contract-relax-reversal-hold-relax

7. _____is the unilateral termination of care without the patient's consent.

    a. Abandonment

    b. Malfeasance

    c. Misfeasance

    d. Implied consent

    e. Abatement

8. _____is a law that allows a spouse or next of kin to give consent for an unresponsive individual.

   a. Expressed consent

   b. Implied consent

   c. Medicolegal judgment

   d. Forcible restraint

   e. Good Samaritan Act

9. Which of the following are diagnostic special tests for thoracic outlet syndrome?

   Choose all that apply.

   a. Roos test

   b. anterior drawer test

   c. O'Brien test

   d. military brace test

   e. piano key test

   f. Adson's test

   g. crossover test

10. A/n_____sternoclavicular dislocation is a potentially life-threatening injury.

   a. anterior

   b. posterior

   c. lateral

   d. medial

   e. all of the above

11. In the diagram below, identify the area of the **spleen**.

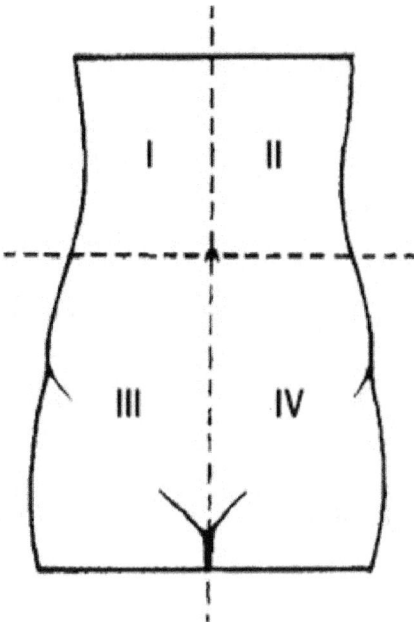

12. _____ is activated and utilized for movements that occur rapidly before sensory feedback has the opportunity to intervene.

   a. Anticipatory control
   b. Closed loop control
   c. Open loop control
   d. Autonomic control
   e. Somatosensory control

13. _____ is the product of mass and acceleration.

   a. Velocity
   b. Momentum
   c. Force
   d. Power
   e. Work

14. Which of the following are tick-borne diseases?

   Choose all that apply.

   a. Rocky Mountain spotted fever

   b. West Nile virus

   c. scarlet fever

   d. smallpox

   e. Lyme disease

   f. chronic wasting disease

15. Commotio cordis occurs during what part of the cardiac electrical cycle?

   a. depolarization phase

   b. plateau phase

   c. resting phase

   d. T wave

   e. repolarization phase

16. _____ is characterized by a collection of blood in the eye's anterior chamber.

   a. Hyphema

   b. Ruptured globe

   c. Conjunctivitis

   d. Detached retina

   e. Macular degeneration

17. _____ is a type of proton pump inhibitor.

   a. Ibuprofen (Motrin)

   b. Acetaminophen (Tylenol)

   c. Omeprazole (Prilosec)

   d. Sertraline (Zoloft)

   e. Metoprolol (Lopresor)

18. Which of the following are classified as electrolytes?

    Choose all that apply.

    a. chloride

    b. riboflavin

    c. biotin

    d. sodium

    e. sulfur

19. This type of contraction occurs when a muscle generates force while it is changing

    length.

    a. isometric

    b. isokinetic

    c. isotonic

    d. static

    e. all of the above

20. Which of the following is a suffix for antifungal medications?

    a. -cillin

    b. -sone

    c. -azole

    d. -lone

    e. -vir

21. Which of the following would be a rehabilitation technique for treating flat low-back

    posture?

    a. hamstring flexibility

    b. lumbar extensions

    c. hip flexor strengthening

    d. intercostal flexibility

    e. all of the above

22. An athlete is diagnosed with a musculocutaneous nerve injury. Which of the following movements will be affected by this injury?

Choose all that apply.

a. elbow flexion

b. elbow extension

c. forearm pronation

d. shoulder flexion

e. shoulder extension

f. forearm supination

g. thumb extension

23. _____is a skin condition characterized by localized edema and itching that occurs with brief exposure to cold temperatures.

a. Frostnip

b. Frostbite

c. Hypothermia

d. Erythema

e. Cold urticaria

24. It is recommended that athletes should be acclimatized to environmental heat over a period of _____ days.

a. 1-2

b. 4-7

c. 7-14

d. 30-48

e. 60-70

25. An athlete experiencing exertional sickling may show which of the following signs and/or symptoms?

    a. pain

    b. muscle hardness

    c. muscle fatigue

    d. muscle twinges/cramps

    e. all of the above

26. How long are you supposed to hold an EpiPen® in position to deliver the medication?

    a. 5 seconds

    b. 10 seconds

    c. 15 seconds

    d. 20 seconds

    e. 30 seconds

27. Which of the following is a diagnostic special test for medial synovial plica?

    a. patellar apprehension test

    b. sweep test

    c. Wilson's test

    d. Noble test

    e. stutter test

28. Which of the following are signs/symptoms of anorexia athletica?
    Choose all that apply.

    a. binging and purging food

    b. laxative use

    c. excess physical activity

    d. starvation

    e. distorted body image

    f. can be fatal

29. _____is the medical term for bright red blood that is produced by a cough.

    a. Hemoptysis

    b. Hematuria

    c. Hematemesis

    d. Hematochezia

    e. hematopoiesis

30._____refers to black foul-smelling stool.

    a. Diarrhea

    b. Hematochezia

    c. Melena

    d. Hematemesis

    e. Piles

31._____is an infection of the airway below the vocal cords.

    a. Upper respiratory infection

    b. Bronchitis

    c. Croup

    d. Sinusitis

    e. All of the above

32. _____are crackling breath sounds that are caused by narrowed airways.

    a. Stridor

    b. Wheezing

    c. Rales

    d. Rhonchi

    e. Croup

33. A patient with a hyphema should be placed in a/n_____position until further treatment
is available.

    a. fully supine

    b. fully prone

    c. recumbent or semi-recumbent

    d. standing

    e. seated

34. Which of the following is the most appropriate tool for definitively diagnosing a corneal
abrasion?

    a. Snellen chart

    b. fluorescein drops and fluorescent light

    c. photosensitivity test

    d. computed tomography

    e. visual acuity test

35. Which of the following are diagnostic special tests for biceps tendonitis?
    Choose all that apply.

    a. Hawkins-Kennedy test

    b. Yergason's test

    c. Speed's test

    d. Neer's test

    e. Adson's test

    f. Allen's test

36. Soft tissue's adaptation to submaximal demands is known as_____.

    a. Wolff's law

    b. Davis's law

    c. Hooke's law

    d. Charles's law

    e. All of the above

37. _____ is a chemical that increases the permeability of blood vessels.

    a. Neutrophil

    b. Histamine

    c. Phagocyte

    d. Leukocyte

    e. Cortisol

38. A 28-year-old male is training for an Ironman Triathlon and has decided to focus on cycling by dramatically increasing his time on the bicycle. He has also chosen a new type of saddle (seat) that is lighter but contains significantly less cushioning than the previous one. He experiences pain in the lower gluteal area immediately following his long training rides. Based on the information given, what would be the most likely injury?

    a. ischial bursitis

    b. trochanteric bursitis

    c. snapping hip syndrome

    d. Legg-Calve-Perthes disease

    e. SI joint dysfunction

39. Which of the following is an effective ankle stretch position for a plantar fasciitis night splint?

    a. 25° of plantarflexion

    b. 50° of plantarflexion

    c. neutral position

    d. 5° of dorsiflexion

    e. 20° of dorsiflexion

40. Hypertrophic cardiomyopathy is an enlargement of what cardiac structure(s)?

    a. aortic valve

    b. aorta

    c. mitral valve

    d. coronary arteries

    e. interventricular septum/left ventricle

41. The greatest concern when dealing with a deep vein thrombosis is that it can

    cause a/n_____.

    a. pulmonary embolism

    b. amputation

    c. aortic aneurysm

    d. aortic dissection

    e. myocardial infarction

42. Corticosteroids are notorious for which side effect?

    a. fatigue

    b. angioedema

    c. cough

    d. increased blood glucose

    e. hyponatremia

43._____is a bacterial skin infection characterized by raised blisters that rupture to create a

    honey-colored crust.

    a. Tinea corporis

    b. Impetigo

    c. Folliculitis

    d. Molluscum contagiosum

    e. Herpes simplex

44. Lightning procedures should be complete and danger is imminent when lightning is

    within_____.

    a. 6 miles

    b. 10 miles

    c. 15 miles

    d. 20 miles

    e. 25 miles

45. Which of the following are signs and symptoms of hyponatremia?

   Choose all that apply.

   a. acute weight loss

   b. acute weight gain

   c. altered mental status

   d. diarrhea

   e. seizure

   f. cramping

46. _____is a congenital deformity characterized by an underdeveloped scapula that sits

   high on the posterior aspect of the thorax.

   a. Stener lesion

   b. Sprengel's deformity

   c. Thoracic outlet syndrome

   d. Scapular winging

   e. Hooked acromion

47. _____is a congenital condition characterized by the incomplete closure of the posterior

   lamina of the lumbar spine.

   a. Spina bifida occulta

   b. Scoliosis

   c. Scheuermann's disease

   d. Ankylosing spondylitis

   e. Lumbarization

48. _____is the process of utilizing the body's innate mechanisms in order to rid a wound

   of necrotic tissue.

   a. Healing

   b. Autolytic debridement

   c. Wound bedding

   d. Autogranulation

   e. Wet-to-dry debridement

49. Following a tooth avulsion, which of the following is the most proper method of preserving the tooth until referral to a specialist is achieved?

a. Immerse the tooth in saline solution.

b. Immerse the tooth in milk.

c. Rinse the tooth with saline and hold it against the tongue.

d. Rinse the tooth with saline and place it back in the socket.

e. Wrap the tooth in gauze and place in ice.

50. The recommended dietary protein intake for a strength athlete is_____.

a. 0.9-1 g/kg of body weight

b. 1.2-1.4 g/kg of body weight

c. 1.5-1.7 g/kg of body weight

d. 1.7-1.8 g/kg of body weight

e. 2.0-2.4 g/kg of body weight

Matching Section (Simulates Drag and Drop)

Match the term on the left with its corresponding description.

Questions 51-55

Topic: Heat Illness

51.____heat exhaustion   a. hot, red, and dry skin

52.____heat stroke   b. caused by heat and friction

53.____heat cramps   c. cool and clammy skin

54.____heat syncope   d. occurs due to electrolyte imbalance

55.____heat rash   e. caused by excess standing and heat

56. What is used to lift a foreign body off of the eye?

   a. gloved finger

   b. hypodermic needle

   c. tweezers

   d. sterile cotton swab

   e. sterile tongue depressor

57. Which of the following are causes of acute conjunctivitis?

   Choose all that apply.

   a. bacteria

   b. virus

   c. genetics

   d. medication

   e. fungus

   f. asthma

58. The_____is upheld by using what a reasonably prudent person with similar training and experience would do in a similar circumstance.

   a. duty

   b. standard of care

   c. code of ethics

   d. medical practices act

   e. all of the above

59. _____is unlawfully placing a person in fear of immediate bodily harm without consent.

   a. Assault

   b. Battery

   c. False imprisonment

   d. Kidnapping

   e. Negligence

60. _____The nerve roots that supply the common fibular (peroneal) nerve are_____.

    a. L1-L4

    b. L3-S1

    c. L4-S3

    d. S1-S3

    e. L1-S3

Matching Section (Simulates Drag and Drop)

Match the term on the left with its appropriate description on the right.

Questions 61-68

Topic: Cranial Nerves

61._____olfactory   a. vision

62._____optic   b. face movements

63._____spinal accessory   c. face sensation

64._____vagus   d. parasympathetic nervous system function

65._____trigeminal   e. tongue movement

66._____hypoglossal   f. lateral eye movement

67._____facial   g. shoulder elevation

68._____abducens   h. smell

69. The amount and distribution of buoyancy for aquatic therapy is determined by_____.

    a. lean mass

    b. distribution of fat

    c. amount of air in chest

    d. gender

    e. all of the above

70. Which of the following are classified as accessory motions of joints?

   Choose all that apply.

   a. glide

   b. distraction

   c. flexion

   d. abduction

   e. adduction

   f. extension

   g. circumduction

   h. compression

71. Which of the following is pes cavus a contributing factor to?

   a. plantar fasciitis

   b. genu valgum

   c. hammer toe

   d. Achilles pathology

   e. all of the above

72. Which of the following is a closed kinetic chain exercise for the lower extremity?

   a. short-arc quad exercises (SAQ)

   b. prone hamstring curls

   c. terminal knee extensions (TKE)

   d. quad sets

   e. all of the above

73. Which of the following structures is the most frequently injured?

   a. anterior cruciate ligament

   b. posterior cruciate ligament

   c. medial collateral ligament

   d. lateral collateral ligament

   e. arcuate ligament

74. A 13-year-old female gymnast is complaining of a backache. Upon observation, there is visible hyperkyphosis of the thoracic spine. There is palpable point tenderness on the spinous processes of T10-L2. Diagnostic imaging reveals decreased space between the thoracic segments with associated degeneration of the vertebral body endplates. Based on the information given, what would be the likely cause of these signs/symptoms?

a. facet joint dysfunction

b. spondylolisthesis

c. spondylolysis

d. Scheuermann's disease

e. wedge fracture

75. This term describes when consecutive ribs are fractured and they move back towards inspiration and forward during expiration.

a. flail chest

b. traumatic pneumothorax

c. sucking chest wound

d. floating fracture

e. Chopart fracture

76. If 10 clinicians perform a Lachman test on an athlete with all finding a positive result, what is true of this scenario?

a. high positive likelihood ratio

b. high chance of false positive

c. high chance of true positive

d. high inter-rater reliability

e. high negative likelihood ratio

77. Brachial artery occlusion that inhibits circulation to the forearm, wrist, and hand can result in a/n_____.

   a. ape hand

   b. Volkmann's contracture

   c. Dupuytren's contracture

   d. Gilliat-Sumner hand

   e. all of the above

78. _____is a benign collection of fluid within a tendinous sheath or joint capsule in the wrist or hand.

   a. Ganglion cyst

   b. Sebaceous cyst

   c. Baker's cyst

   d. Carpal cyst

   e. Pilonidal cyst

79. Hyporeflexia of the Achilles tendon is indicative of which nerve root injury?

   a. L1-L2

   b. L2-L3

   c. L4-L5

   d. S1-S2

   e. S2-S3

80. _____is a defect on the anterior aspect of the humeral head.

   a. Bankart lesion

   b. Reverse Bankart lesion

   c. Hill-Sachs lesion

   d. Reverse Hill-Sachs lesion

   e. SLAP lesion

End of Exam 1

Exam 1 Answers/Domains

1. a. I	41. a. III
2. c. II	42. d. IV
3. b. II	43. b. II
4. a. III	44. a. I
5. b. IV	45. b. c. e. I
6. c. IV	46. b. I
7. a. V	47. a. I
8. c. V	48. b. IV
9. a. d. f. II	49. d. IV
10. b. II	50. d. I
11. upper left quadrant. I	51. c. I
12. c. I	52. a. I
13. c. I	53. d. I
14. a. e. II	54. e. I
15. e. III	55. b. I
16. a. II	56. d. IV
17. c. IV	57. a. b. II
18. a. d. I	58. b. V
19. c. I	59. a. V
20. c. IV	60. c. I
21. e. IV	61. h. I
22. a. d. f. II	62. a. I
23. e. I	63. g. I
24. c. I	64. d. I
25. e. III	65. c. I
26. b. III	66. e. I
27. e. II	67. b. I
28. c. e. f. I	68. f. I
29. a. II	69. e. IV
30. c. II	70. a. b. c. I
31. c. II	71. c. II
32. c. II	72. c. IV
33. c. IV	73. c. II
34. b. II	74. d. II
35. b. c. II	75. a. III
36. b. I	76. d. I
37. b. IV	77. b. II
38. a. II	78. a. II
39. d. IV	79. d. II
40. e. I	80. d. II

Exam 2 on Next Page

Exam 2

80 questions

4 hour maximum

1. An exercise where resistance is provided at a fixed velocity with accommodating resistance is known as_____.
   a. isotonic
   b. concentric
   c. eccentric
   d. isokinetic
   e. isometric

2. _____is a type of non-steroidal anti-inflammatory drug.
   a. Sertraline (Zoloft)
   b. Prednisone
   c. Cortisone
   d. Acetaminophen (Tylenol)
   e. Naproxen (Aleve)

3. _____is a type of budget where items are separated into categories with a set amount of funds assigned to each.
   a. Lump-sum
   b. Line-item
   c. Fixed
   d. Zero-based
   e. Spending-ceiling model

4. _____is a condition that results from vitamin D deficiency.
   a. Scurvy
   b. Rickets
   c. Beriberi
   d. Pellagra
   e. Xerophthalmia

5. _____is a condition that results from vitamin C deficiency.

    a. Scurvy

    b. Rickets

    c. Beriberi

    d. Pellagra

    e. Xerophthalmia

6. _____is responsible for football helmet certification.

    a. NATA

    b. SGMA

    c. CSA

    d. NOCSAE

    e. NAIA

7. What is characterized by a fracture of the base of the first metacarpal bone?

    a. Colles' fracture

    b. Smith's fracture

    c. Bennett's fracture

    d. Jones fracture

    e. boxer's fracture

8. _____is fluid that escapes from the blood vessels into the adjacent tissue.

    a. Exudate

    b. Extravasate

    c. Edema

    d. Ecchymosis

    e. All of the above

9. _____is the most common site on the clavicle for a fracture to occur.

   a. The distal 1/3rd

   b. The middle 1/3rd

   c. The proximal 1/3rd

10. Which of the following movements would you test for C7's myotome?

    Choose all that apply.

    a. Wrist extension

    b. Wrist flexion

    c. Wrist radial deviation

    d. Wrist ulnar deviation

    e. Elbow flexion

    f. Elbow extension

    g. Shoulder flexion

11. _____is characterized as an inferior glenohumeral ligament avulsion with a labral tear

    following a dislocation.

    a. Bankart lesion

    b. Reverse Bankart lesion

    c. Hill-Sachs lesion

    d. Reverse Hill-Sachs lesion

    e. SLAP lesion

12. _____is responsible for ice hockey helmet certification.

    a. NATA

    b. SGMA

    c. CSA

    d. NOCSAE

    e. NAIA

13. Which of the following are classified as fat soluble vitamins?

    Choose all that apply.

    a. thiamin

    b. vitamin K

    c. niacin

    d. vitamin C

    e. vitamin E

    f. riboflavin

    g. pantothenic acid

    h. folic acid

14. _____is an injury to the posterior humeral head's articular cartilage, and is caused by impact of the humeral head on the glenoid when an attempt at reduction is made.

    a. Bankart lesion

    b. Reverse Bankart lesion

    c. Hill-Sachs lesion

    d. Reverse Hill-Sachs lesion

    e. SLAP lesion

15. The painful arc between 70°-120° of shoulder abduction is associated with_____.

    a. rotator cuff tendinopathy

    b. thoracic outlet syndrome

    c. impingement

    d. brachial plexus neuropraxia

    e. anterior glenohumeral instability

16. _____states that pressure exerted by fluid on an immersed object is equal on the whole area of the object.

    a. Boyle's law

    b. Bernoulli's principle

    c. Pascal's law

    d. Newton's 3rd law of motion

    e. Avogadro's law

17. Two months after surgery to repair a female athlete's patellar tendon, her scar was starting to limit her knee mobility. Which of the following is the most appropriate treatment?

    a. petrissage

    b. effleurage

    c. friction massage

    d. tapotement

    e. myofascial release

18. Sensory information ascending the spinal cord is routed to its designated location in the brain by the_____.

    a. pons

    b. cerebellum

    c. medulla oblongata

    d. thalamus

    e. cerebrum

19. This ligament prevents the radius from dislocating and sliding distally.

    a. RCL

    b. LUCL

    c. LCL

    d. arcuate ligament

    e. annular ligament

20. This ligament provides rotary stability for the elbow joint.

    a. RCL

    b. LUCL

    c. LCL

    d. arcuate ligament

    e. annular ligament

21. _____is the most appropriate diagnostic test for a high ankle sprain.

    a. Anterior drawer

    b. Homan's sign

    c. Eversion stress test

    d. Kleiger's test

    e. Bump test

22. Most deaths due to lightning strikes occur as a result of_____.

    a. severe burns

    b. shock

    c. tissue injury

    d. cardiac arrest

    e. respiratory arrest

23. Which of the following is a special test for an acromioclavicular sprain?

    a. anterior drawer test

    b. Phalen's test

    c. clunk test

    d. Adson's test

    e. piano key sign

24. Which of the following are signs/symptoms of anorexia nervosa?

    Choose all that apply.

    a. hunger denial

    b. binging and purging food

    c. excess physical activity

    d. tooth decay

    e. stomach rupture

    f. esophageal erosion

25. Kicking a ball is an example of a/n_____activity.

    a. open kinetic chain

    b. closed kinetic chain

    c. static

    d. unskilled

    e. simple

26. _____is the term for when a patient experiences a continuous seizure without a lucid period for at least 30 minutes.

   a. Postictal period

   b. Grand mal

   c. Petit mal

   d. Status epilepticus

   e. Tonic-clonic

27._____are small raised areas of itching or burning as a result of an allergic reaction.

   a. Urticaria

   b. Vitiligo

   c. Cellulitis

   d. Macules

   e. Pustules

28. Unusually frequent drinking of water in fluids to satisfy thirst in diabetic individuals is called_____.

   a. urticaria

   b. polyuria

   c. polydipsia

   d. polyphagia

   e. polycystitis

29. An infection of an eyelash follicle is known as _____.

   a. stye

   b. acute conjunctivitis

   c. blepharitis

   d. scleroderma

   e. follicular abscess

30. Which of the following are diagnostic special tests for subacromial impingement?

   Choose all that apply.

   a. Neer's test

   b. Speed's test

   c. Adson's test

   d. Allen's test

   e. military brace test

   f. Hawkins-Kennedy test

31. The dermatome of the _____ is located on the lateral forearm, and its myotome is tested with elbow flexion.

   a. axillary nerve

   b. musculocutaneous nerve

   c. radial nerve

   d. ulnar nerve

   e. spinal accessory nerve

32. _____is the initial type of collagen that is introduced to an injured tissue during the proliferation phase before it is replaced with a more refined type of collagen.

   a. Type I

   b. Type II

   c. Type III

   d. Type IV

   e. Type V

33. A 25-year-old male athlete presents in the athletic training room with a bump on the posterior aspect of the heel. It is red, inflamed, and painful to the touch. The athlete states that it has been there for a while, but the new shoes he is wearing have irritated it. What is the likely injury/condition?

    a. sever's disease

    b. os trigonum

    c. achilles tendonitis

    d. plantar calcaneal exostosis

    e. Haglund's deformity

34. _____ is the rapid structural breakdown of muscle tissue due to lack of blood supply.

    a. Exertional rhabdomyolysis

    b. Metabolic acidosis

    c. Acute mountain sickness

    d. Acute ischemic rhabdomyolysis

    e. Hypoxemia

35. Which of the following would be plyometric exercises when rehabilitating an ACL reconstruction?

    Choose all that apply.

    a. tuck jump

    b. hip bridge

    c. shuttle run

    d. scissor jump

    e. butt kickers

    f. carioca

    g. ankle bounce

36. _____ is a bacterial infection that usually occurs on skin that has been recently shaved, taped, or abraded. The patient presents with papules and pustules at the base of hair follicles.

   a. Impetigo
   b. Folliculitis
   c. Ingrown hair
   d. Cellulitis
   e. Molluscum contagiosum

37. Which of the following medications is indicated when an athlete is experiencing an acute asthma episode?

   Choose all that apply.

   a. $\square_2$-agonist
   b. aspirin
   c. exercise
   d. corticosteroids
   e. NSAID
   f. proton-pump inhibitor

38. Which of the following are first aid procedures following a lightning strike?
   Choose all that apply.
   a. Beware of a residual electric charge on the victim.
   b. Activate EMS.
   c. Initiate CPR if necessary.
   d. Never move the victim.
   e. Administer pain medication.
   f. Treat for dehydration.

39. _____occurs when there is inflammation of a bony projection that serves as a muscle attachment.
    a. Apophysitis
    b. Myositis
    c. Periostitis
    d. Tendinosis
    e. Tenosynovitis

40. _____is characterized by an acute spasm of digital blood vessels in response to emotional distress or cold exposure.
    a. Frostnip
    b. Frostbite
    c. Raynaud's syndrome
    d. Cold urticaria
    e. Hypothermia

41. The depth of penetration for therapeutic ultrasound while using 1MHz frequency is_____.
    a. 1 cm
    b. 2 cm
    c. 3 cm
    d. 4 cm
    e. 5 cm

42. An athlete presents with spasms of the left strernocleidomastoid muscle and his chin is rotated to the right side. What is the most likely condition?
    a. thoracic outlet syndrome
    b. cervical disc herniation
    c. torticollis
    d. facet joint dysfunction
    e. meningitis

43. A 23 year old male baseball pitcher presents with shoulder pain during the follow-through of his pitching motion during a bullpen session. Which of the following would be the most likely cause?

a. SLAP lesion

b. pectoralis major strain

c. thoracic outlet syndrome

d. acromioclavicular sprain

e. Hill-Sachs lesion

44. A disorder to which structure of the ear would be most likely to cause vertigo?

a. cochlea

b. semicircular canals

c. tympanic membrane

d. stapes

e. auricle

45. A 12-year-old athlete sustained a supracondylar fracture 14 months ago. She didn't require surgery, and was casted. She is now experiencing pain and inflammation with cubitus varus. What is the most likely cause?

a. lateral epicondylitis

b. medial epicondylitis

c. nonunion fracture and gunstock deformity

d. Volkmann's contracture

e. osteochondritis dissecans

46. Which of the following spinal conditions would cause a sudden loss of bladder and/or bowel function?

a. thoracic outlet syndrome

b. brachial plexus neuropraxia

c. cauda equina syndrome

d. fractured coccyx

e. all of the above

Matching Section (Simulates Drag and Drop)

Match the term on the left with its corresponding description.

Questions 47-54

Topic: Fractures

47._____Jones fracture   a. fracture/dislocation of midfoot

48._____Bennett's fracture   b. common wrist fracture in juveniles

49._____Galeazzi fracture   c. distal radius fracture with volar displacement

50._____Monteggia fracture   d. 5th metacarpal fracture

51._____buckle fracture   e. fracture of the base of the thumb

52._____Smith fracture   f. distal radius fracture with distal radioulnar dx.

53._____boxer's fracture   g. proximal ulna fracture with radial head dx.

54._____Lisfranc fracture   h. base of the 5th metatarsal fracture

55. Which of the following is the most appropriate medication for treatment of acute
    conjunctivitis?

    a. acetaminophen (Tylenol)

    b. ibuprofen (Motrin)

    c. naproxen sodium (Aleve)

    d. Acyclovir

    e. sulfacetamide

56. The lumbar plexus is supplied by nerve roots_____.

    a. T6-T12

    b. T8-L3

    c. T10-L2

    d. T12-L4

    e. L5-S3

57. Which of the following muscles are innervated by the median nerve?

Choose all that apply.

a. triceps brachii

b. biceps brachii

c. palmaris longus

d. brachialis

e. flexor carpi radialis

f. extensor pollicis brevis

g. pronator quadratus

58. Which position places the least amount of stress on the lumbar spine?

a. extension

b. flexion

c. anterior pelvic tilt

d. pelvic neutral

e. posterior pelvic tilt

59. Which of the following is an example of a vector for communicable disease transmission?

a. air

b. surface

c. water

d. mosquito

e. all of the above

60. _____ has guidelines that require all employees to be afforded a work environment with minimal exposure to hazards.

a. OSHA

b. CDC

c. NFPA

d. NATA

e. FMLA

Matching Section (Simulates Drag and Drop)

Match the term on the left with its corresponding description.

Questions 61-63

Topic: Hepatitis

61._____Hepatitis A   a. blood or sexual contact

62._____Hepatitis B   b. fecal matter or infected food

63._____Hepatitis C   c. blood, saliva, urine or breast milk

64. Special testing would be documented in what section of SOAP?

   a. S

   b. O

   c. A

   d. P

   e. both a. and b.

65._____is a serious condition that includes pregnancy-induced hypertension and usually occurs after the 20th

   week of pregnancy.

   a. Supine hypotensive syndrome

   b. Pre-eclampsia

   c. Placenta previa

   d. Hyperemesis gravidarum

   e. Polyhydramnios

66. In the diagram below, identify the location of the descending colon.

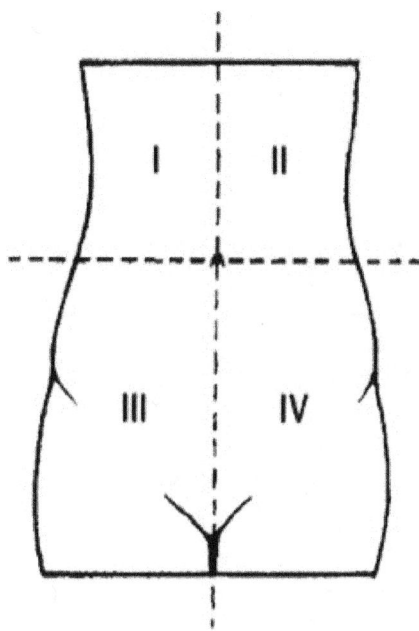

67._____is the ability to utilize diet, sleep, activity, and medicine in order to achieve

positive health outcomes.

   a. Emotional wellness

   b. Intellectual wellness

   c. Physical wellness

   d. Spiritual wellness

   e. Occupational wellness

68._____is a psychological condition characterized by alternating bouts of mania and

depression.

   a. Obsessive compulsive disorder

   b. Dissociative disorder

   c. Bipolar disorder

   d. Anxiety disorder

   e. Schizophrenia

69. The log-roll technique requires a minimum of_____rescuers in order to be accomplished in a safe manner.

   a. 1-2
   b. 2-3
   c. 3-4
   d. 4-5
   e. 5-6

70. Following an injury, active range of motion_____.

   a. promotes hematoma absorption
   b. increases tensile-strength
   c. promotes myofibril regeneration
   d. improves collagen arrangement
   e. all of the above

71._____is the ability of tissue to return to normal length after being lengthened due to a force being applied.

   a. Elasticity
   b. Viscosity
   c. Viscoelasticity
   d. Plasticity
   e. Extensibility

72. The presence of a cervical rib predisposes an individual to develop_____.

   a. cervical nerve root compression
   b. impingement
   c. thoracic outlet syndrome
   d. brachial plexus neuropraxia
   e. all of the above

73. The_____is formed by a widening of the supraspinous ligament in the cervical spine.

   a. interspinous ligament

   b. ligamentum nuchae

   c. ligamentum flavum

   d. tectorial membrane

   e. atlanto-occipital ligament

74. _____is a condition characterized by the L5 and S1 segments fusing together.

   a. Lumbarization

   b. Sacralization

   c. SI joint dysfunction

   d. Pott's disease

   e. Spinal fusion

75. Which of the following is the appropriate progression for a water rescue?

   a. throw and tow, row, go, then reach

   b. reach, throw and tow, go, then row

   c. reach, throw and tow, row, then go

   d. row, throw and tow, reach, then go

   e. row, reach, throw and tow, then go

76. _____is a hormone that allows glucose to enter the body's cells.

   a. Estrogen

   b. Testosterone

   c. Insulin

   d. Vitamin D

   e. hCG

77. _____ is the first cardiac structure that receives oxygenated blood from the pulmonary vein.

   a. Right atrium

   b. Left atrium

   c. Right ventricle

   d. Left ventricle

   e. Aorta

78. What structure is the most common source of epistaxis?

   a. Kiesselbach's plexus

   b. facial artery

   c. supraorbital artery

   d. angular artery

   e. carotid sinus

79. _____ is a special test utilized for revealing sciatic nerve pathology.

   a. Bilateral straight leg raise test

   b. Well straight leg raise test

   c. Unilateral straight leg raise test

   d. Sitting root test

   e. All of the above

80. _____ is a special test utilized for revealing SI joint dysfunction.

   a. SI joint compression test

   b. Gaenslen's test

   c. FABER test

   d. Bilateral straight leg raise test

   e. All of the above

End of Exam 2

Exam 2 Answers/Domains

1. d. IV	41. e. IV
2. e. IV	42. c. II
3. b. V	43. a. II
4. b. I	44. b. I
5. a. I	45. c. II
6. d. I	46. c. II
7. c. II	47. h. II
8. b. II	48. e. II
9. a. II	49. f. II
10. b. f. I	50. g. II
11. a. II	51. b. II
12. d. I	52. c. II
13. b. e. I	53. d. II
14. c. II	54. a. II
15. c. II	55. e. IV
16. c. IV	56. d. I
17. c. IV	57. c. e. g. I
18. d. I	58. d. I
19. e. I	59. d. I
20. b. I	60. a. V
21. d. II	61. b. I
22. d. III	62. c. I
23. e. II	63. a. I
24. a. c. I	64. b. V
25. a. IV	65. b. I
26. d. III	66. lower left quadrant I
27. a. II	67. c. I
28. c. I	68. c. I
29. c. II	69. d. III
30. a. f. II	70. e. IV
31. b. I	71. a. IV
32. c. IV	72. c. II
33. e. II	73. b. I
34. d. III	74. b. I
35. a. d. g. IV	75. c. III
36. b. II	76. c. I
37. a. d. IV	77. b. I
38. b. c. III	78. a. II
39. a. II	79. d. II
40. c. I	80. e. II

Exam 3 on next page

Exam 3

80 questions

4 hour maximum

1. Which of the following would be a contraindication for taking NSAIDs?

    a. kidney disease

    b. GI ulceration

    c. cardiovascular disease

    d. diabetes

    e. all of the above

2. Somatotropin, also known as_____, is a polypeptide hormone.

    a. anabolic-androgenic steroids

    b. corticosteroids

    c. testosterone

    d. estrogen

    e. human growth hormone

3. _____are drugs that promote the excretion of sodium and chloride ions.

    a. Diuretics

    b. Antipyretics

    c. Anticholinergics

    d. Antiemetic

    e. Anti-inflammatories

4. Ankle dorsiflexion is provided by which myotome?

    a. L3

    b. L4

    c. L5

    d. S1

    e. S2

5. Irregular gasping or shallow breathing that is a common sign of impending cardiac arrest is known as_____.

   a. rhonchi

   b. rales

   c. agonal breathing

   d. bradypnea

   e. tachypnea

6. What category of shock is caused by a sudden dilation of blood vessels?

   a. psychogenic

   b. cardiogenic

   c. neurogenic

   d. hyperthermic

   e. hypothermic

7. Which of the following are signs and/or symptoms of shock?

   Choose all that apply.

   a. excessive thirst

   b. loss of consciousness

   c. red skin

   d. shivering

   e. bradycardia

8. A general estimate of a 30 year old individual's maximum heart rate is_____.

   a. 160 beats per minute

   b. 170 beats per minute

   c. 180 beats per minute

   d. 190 beats per minute

   e. 200 beats per minute

9. _____ involves the transfer of heat via the movement of fluid or gasses.

   a. Conduction

   b. Convection

   c. Radiation

   d. Conversion

   e. Evaporation

10. If tissue is exposed to cold between 15-30 minutes, vasodilation then occurs in order to combat tissue damage. What is this process called?

    a. Raynaud's phenomenon

    b. Hunting response

    c. rebound effect

    d. frostnip

11. What section of SOAP would contain the results of the history?

    a. subjective

    b. objective

    c. assessment

    d. plan

    e. (both a. and b.)

12. When a certified athletic trainer is in violation of the standards of care, this is classified as_____.

    a. misfeasance

    b. malfeasance

    c. nonfeasance

    d. presumptive negligence

    e. comparative negligence

13. In order to prove negligence, there must be_____.

    a. intent to cause harm

    b. a criminal case

    c. damages

    d. case law

    e. consent

14. _____represent(s) the most superficial passage of the brachial plexus.

    a. McBurney's point

    b. Erb's point

    c. The subclavicular region

    d. The scalenes

    e. The jugular notch

15. The dose of epinephrine in an EPIPEN JR® is_____.

    a. 0.15mg

    b. 0.30mg

    c. 0.50mg

    d. 1.00mg

    e. 1.50mg

16. Which of the following is a typical symptom of meningitis?

    a. severe headache

    b. photophobia

    c. neck stiffness

    d. fever

    e. all of the above

17. _____is a condition caused by the Epstein-Barr virus and causes symptoms similar to the common cold.

   a. Lyme disease

   b. Rocky Mountain spotted fever

   c. Infectious mononucleosis

   d. Rhinitis

   e. Typhoid fever

18. Which of the following must a practitioner consider before administering aquatic therapy to a patient?

   a. fear of water

   b. respiratory disorder

   c. neurological disorder

   d. G-tubes

   e. all of the above

19. When performing joint mobilizations involving a concave joint member moving on a fixed convex mate, the mobilization should occur in the_____as bony movement.

   a. same direction

   b. opposite direction

20. _____is a thin membrane that lines the entire abdominal cavity.

   a. Fascia

   b. Peritoneum

   c. Diaphragm

   d. Epithelium

   e. Aponeurosis

21. Which of the following is a diagnostic test for supraspinatus tendinopathy?

    a. load and shift test

    b. Speed's test

    c. Yergason's test

    d. empty can test

    e. All of the above

22. _____refers to posture characterized by excessive knee hyperextension.

    a. Genu valgum

    b. Genu varum

    c. Tibial torsion

    d. Genu recurvatum

    e. Patella baja

23. _____is characterized by a flexion contracture of the metacarpophalangeal and

proximal interphalangeal joints.

    a. De Quervain's disease

    b. Trigger finger

    c. Boutonniere deformity

    d. Mallet finger

    e. Dupuytren's contracture

24. What is the best rapid cooling method for an athlete experiencing exertional heat stroke?

    a. sitting in front of an electric fan

    b. laying on a bed of ice

    c. cold-water immersion

    d. intravenous fluids

    e. rapid rehydration

25. Which of the following are signs and/or symptoms of exertional hyponatremia?

   Choose all that apply.

   a. muscular twitching

   b. peripheral swelling

   c. headache

   d. thirst

   e. dry red skin

   f. lucid interval

   g. seizure

   h. exhaustion

   i. insomnia

26. Which of the following are signs/symptoms of upper crossed syndrome?

   Choose all that apply.

   a. inhibited abdominals

   b. inhibited serratus anterior

   c. inhibited pectoralis major

   d. facilitated lower trapezius

   e. facilitated thoraco-lumbar extensors

   f. facilitated iliopsoas

   g. facilitated pectoralis major

27. Which mechanoreceptor is responsible for detecting sensations of vibration?

   a. hair follicles

   b. Meissner corpuscles

   c. Ruffini corpuscles

   d. Pacinian corpuscles

   e. Merkel cells

28. _____ is an inflamed sebaceous gland at the edge of the eyelid.

    a. blepharitis

    b. stye

    c. folliculitis

    d. follicular abscess

    e. acute conjunctivitis

29. A collegiate female volleyball athlete presents with paresthesia on her right posterior lateral arm, lateral forearm, and third finger. Upon further evaluation, she has weakness in elbow extension and wrist flexion when comparing bilaterally. Her triceps reflex is absent. Which nerve root do you suspect is involved?

    a. C5

    b. C6

    c. C7

    d. C8

    e. T1

30. What ultrasound frequency is indicated for treating patellar tendonitis?

    a. 1 MHz

    b. 2 MHz

    c. 3 MHz

    d. 4 MHz

    e. 5 MHz

31. What is a diagnostic special test used for identifying labral pathology in a hip?

    a. quadrant test

    b. Thomas test

    c. FABER test

    d. Ely's test

    e. Renne test

32. _____ is the amount of force required to change the shape and/or length of tissue.

    a. Stress

    b. Strain

    c. Inertia

    d. Momentum

    e. Torque

33. A 33-year-old female professional distance runner is diagnosed with genu valgum and a squinting patella. Which of the following would be a potential cause of these conditions?

    a. snapping hip syndrome

    b. coxa vara

    c. coxa plana

    d. coxa valga

    e. coxa magna

34. _____ is based on a fixed budget but can be adjusted based on revenue.

    a. Line-item

    b. Zero-based

    c. Incremental

    d. Variable

    e. Rollover

35. _____ is a piece of equipment that can be used for alleviating the symptoms of plantar fasciitis.

    a. Heel cup

    b. Aircast

    c. Neoprene sleeve

    d. Open basket weave taping

    e. Hinged ankle brace

36. When acclimating to heat, what football equipment should be worn on the first two days of practice?

    a. helmet

    b. shoulder pads

    c. helmet and shoulder pads

    d. full equipment

    e. no equipment

37. Which of the following is an important step in preventing death caused by exertional sickling?

    a. medication

    b. screening and precautions

    c. avoiding athletic activities

    d. oxygen administration

    e. sleep

Matching Section (Simulates Drag and Drop)

Match the core temperature on the left with its corresponding description.

Questions 38-43

Topic: Hypothermia

38. _____ 96-99°   a. loss of awareness and bradycardia

39. _____ 91-95°   b. cardiac and respiratory arrest

40. _____ 86-90°   c. unconsciousness and absent reflexes

41. _____ 81-85°   d. speech difficulty

42. _____ 78-80°   e. involuntary shivering

43. _____ <78°   f. shivering decreases and muscular spasm

44. Which of the following are innervated by the suprascapular nerve?

   Choose all that apply.

   a. supraspinatus

   b. subscapularis

   c. infraspinatus

   d. teres major

   e. latissimus dorsi

   f. coracobrachialis

45. Which of the following are signs/symptoms of spondylolysis?

   Choose all that apply.

   a. heart-shaped buttocks

   b. long-strided gait

   c. short-strided gait

   d. lumbar hyperkyphosis

   e. lumbar hyperlordosis

   f. thoracic spine pain

46. A collegiate football player was performing underhand chin ups and felt a "pop" with instant pain in the cubital fossa. There is an immediate depression deformity on the distal arm. Elbow flexion is a 2+. What is the most likely injury?

   a. distal biceps rupture

   b. distal triceps rupture

   c. proximal biceps rupture

   d. proximal triceps rupture

   e. brachioradialis rupture

47. For the injury in question 46, what would be a special test to reinforce your findings?

    a. bump test
    b. hook test
    c. varus test
    d. valgus test
    e. all of the above

48. Which of the following would be a proper functional progression for a Grade I lateral ankle sprain?

    a. ankle pumps, BAPS balancing, standing jumps
    b. lateral runs, jumps, BAPS balancing
    c. lunges, ankle pumps, cariocas
    d. hops, ankle pumps, sprints
    e. all of the above

49. This proprioceptive neuromuscular facilitation technique is performed by passively stretching the limb, holding the stretch, having the patient perform an isometric contraction for 6 seconds, and then stretching further.

    a. contract-relax
    b. hold-relax
    c. slow-reversal-hold-relax
    d. hold-contract-relax
    e. contract-relax-hold

50. Which of the following are convex joint surfaces?

   Choose all that apply.

   a. femoral head

   b. tibial plateau

   c. femoral condyle

   d. humeral head

   e. ankle mortise

   f. acetabulum

   g. glenoid fossa

51. _____occurs when the placenta separates prematurely from the uterine wall.

   a. placenta abruptio

   b. ectopic pregnancy

   c. placenta previa

   d. eclampsia

   e. obstructive hydrocephalus

52. The_____is the primary regulator of the body's endocrine glands.

   a. thyroid gland

   b. adrenal gland

   c. thalamus

   d. pituitary

   e. pancreas

53. Which of the following are causes of anisocoria?

Choose all that apply.

   a. congenital condition

   b. depressed brain function

   c. hypertension

   d. hypotension

   e. tachycardia

   f. bradycardia

54. _____is an eye condition that is prevalent in the geriatric population and is characterized by a clouding of the lens with associated vision impairments.

   a. Hyphema

   b. Myopia

   c. Cataract

   d. Myasthenia gravis

   e. Detached retina

55. The picture below depicts what injury?

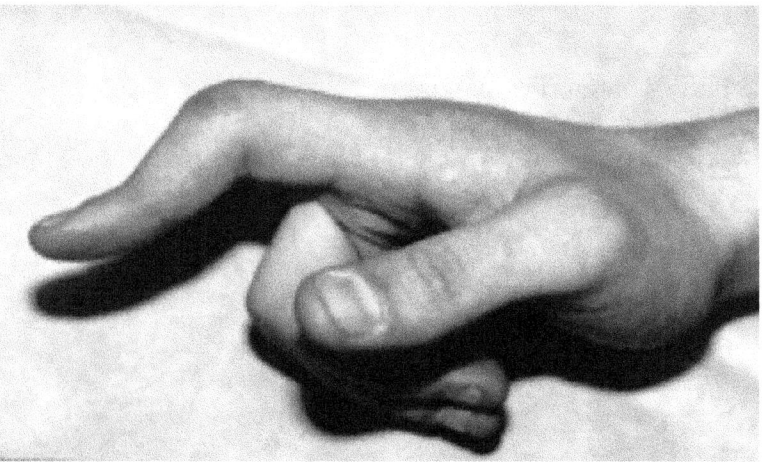

   a. swan neck deformity
   b. trigger finger
   c. mallet finger
   d. boutonniere deformity
   e. jersey finger

Matching Section (Simulates Drag and Drop)

Match the disc injury on the left with its corresponding description.

Questions 56-59

Topic: Disc injuries

56._____protrusion

57._____prolapse

58._____extrusion

59._____sequestration

a. separation of nuclear material

b. herniation to the external border of annulus

c. slight herniation to annulus

d. herniation to middle of annulus

60. _____is a burst fracture of C1 caused by axial loading.

a. Hangman's fracture

b. Jefferson fracture

c. Odontoid fracture

d. Chance fracture

e. Wedge fracture

61._____is the ability to expend resources in order to expand knowledge and skill.

a. Social wellness

b. Emotional wellness

c. Physical wellness

d. Environmental wellness

e. Intellectual wellness

62. _____is a type of budget that allows an increase or decrease only in certain categories based on availability in funds.

a. Line-item

b. Spending-ceiling

c. Balloon

d. Program

e. Zero-based

63. _____ is a type of leadership where the leader goes above and beyond in order to elevate standards and improve the program.
    a. Transactional leadership
    b. Transformational leadership
    c. Transcendent leadership
    d. Charismatic leadership
    e. Authoritarian leadership

64. _____ is a body-regulated state where the optimal amount of body fluid is achieved.
    a. Hyperhydration
    b. Hypohydration
    c. Euhydration
    d. Plasma gradient
    e. Interstitial homeostasis

65. The _____ maneuver is preferred when accessing the airway when there is a suspected traumatic cervical spine injury.
    a. head-tilt
    b. chin-lift
    c. hook and press
    d. jaw-thrust
    e. head rotation

66. _____ occurs in children and is characterized by a flattened capitellum due to avascular necrosis in the elbow.
    a. Little league elbow
    b. Panner's disease
    c. Nursemaid's elbow
    d. Cubital tunnel syndrome
    e. Jones fracture

67. _____ is a condition caused by prolonged sitting.

  a. Greater trochanteric bursitis

  b. Iliopectineal bursitis

  c. Ischiogluteal bursitis

  d. Lumbarization

  e. SI joint dysfunction

68. What position should be avoided if an athlete is in a rehabilitation protocol for posterior glenohumeral instability?

  a. quadruped position

  b. anatomical position

  c. tailor's position

  d. neutral shoulder position

  e. braced position

69. This condition is prevalent in women over 30 years of age on the non-dominant shoulder. This condition usually resolves on its own within 18-24 months.

  a. rotator cuff tendinopathy

  b. adhesive capsulitis

  c. external impingement

  d. gross internal rotation deficit

  e. thoracic outlet syndrome

70. An athlete with a positive lift-off test is most likely to have sustained a/n_____.

  a. supraspinatus tendinopathy

  b. thoracic outlet syndrome

  c. subscapularis tendinopathy

  d. acromioclavicular sprain

  e. sternoclavicular sprain

71. _____ is the primary function of the transversus abdominis.
    a. Trunk flexion
    b. Lateral flexion
    c. Inspiration
    d. Expiration
    e. Compression of abdominal viscera

72. _____ is the location inside or outside of the body where all matter is equally distributed around it.
    a. Base of support
    b. Surface center
    c. Center of gravity
    d. Center of inertia
    e. All of the above

73. Which of the following is the best strategy to develop coordination?
    a. simple to complex
    b. static to dynamic
    c. repetition
    d. increase speed and complexity
    e. all of the above

74. Following an injury, what is the effect of immobilization on muscle tissue?
    a. increased oxidative capacity
    b. increased capillary density
    c. increase in fatty tissue
    d. increased number of myofibrils
    e. all of the above

75. _____ is the amount of force required to change the shape or form of a tissue.

    a. Stress

    b. Strain

    c. Creep

    d. Force-couple

    e. Plasticity

76. Following a venomous pit viper bite, which of the following should be done for immediate treatment?

    Choose all that apply.

    a. apply ice

    b. calm patient

    c. mark bite area with pen

    d. don't clean the area

    e. administer NSAIDs

77. _____ is a disorder that affects the connective tissues, and those affected are usually tall, thin, and susceptible to cardiac issues.

    a. Lupus

    b. Pott's disease

    c. Marfan syndrome

    d. Cystic fibrosis

    e. Fanconi anemia

78. _____ is an abnormal posture characterized by extended knees, flexed wrists, flexed fingers, and extended elbows.

    a. Decorticate

    b. Decerebrate

    c. Dystonia

    d. Myoclonus

    e. Flaccid

79. Decompression sickness occurs when_____bubbles infiltrate the blood vessels.

    a. oxygen gas

    b. helium gas

    c. nitrogen gas

    d. carbon dioxide

    e. carbon monoxide

80. Which of the following special tests is used in order to identify cervical nerve root compression?

    a. flexion test

    b. Spurling test

    c. Froment's sign

    d. Phalen's test

    e. all of the above

End of Exam 3

Exam 3 Answers/Domains

1. d. IV	41. a. I
2. e. I	42. c. I
3. a. IV	43. b. I
4. b. I	44. a. c. I
5. c. III	45. a. c. e. II
6. c. III	46. a. II
7. a. b. III	47. b. II
8. d. I	48. a. IV
9. b. I	49. b. IV
10. b. IV	50. a. c. d. I
11. a. V	51. a. I
12. d. V	52. d. I
13. c. V	53. a. b. III
14. b. I	54. c. I
15. a. III	55. d. II
16. e. III	56. c. II
17. c. I	57. b. II
18. e. IV	58. d. II
19. a. IV	59. a. II
20. b. I	60. b. III
21. d. II	61. e. I
22. d. II	62. b. V
23. e. II	63. b. V
24. c. III	64. c. I
25. a. b. c. g. III	65. d. III
26. b. g. II	66. b. II
27. d. I	67. c. II
28. b. II	68. a. IV
29. c. II	69. b. II
30. c. IV	70. c. II
31. a. II	71. e. I
32. b. I	72. c. I
33. b. II	73. e. I
34. d. V	74. c. IV
35. a. IV	75. a. IV
36. a. I	76. b. c. III
37. b. III	77. c. I
38. e. I	78. b. III
39. d. I	79. c. I
40. f. I	80. b. II

Exam 4 on next page

Exam 4

80 questions

4 hour maximum

1. A tall thin male athlete presents to the training room complaining of non-traumatic unilateral chest pain and shortness of breath. You listen to his lungs and do not hear any breath sounds on the right side. What condition are you concerned about?
   a. pulmonary embolism
   b. pneumothorax
   c. orthostatic hypotension
   d. commotio cordis
   e. cardiac tamponade

2. _____is the leading cause of death within the first 24 hours following injury in sports.
   a. Commotio cordis
   b. Hypertrophic cardiomyopathy
   c. Subdural hematoma
   d. Second impact syndrome
   e. Rhabdomyolysis

3. Which of the following are signs and/or symptoms of concussions?
   Choose all that apply.
   a. mental fog
   b. lucidity
   c. enhanced reaction time
   d. amnesia
   e. cognitive fog

4. Which of the following conditions is a concern between 3-6 weeks post mononucleosis infection?

   a. myocardial infarction

   b. spleen rupture

   c. jaundice

   d. exertional sickling

   e. rhabdomyolysis

5. _____occur due to a collagen disease that affects the body's connective tissue.

   a. Cafe'-au-lait spots

   b. Vitiligo

   c. Spina bifida occulta

   d. Scheuermann's disease

   e. All of the above

6. Mild hypothermia begins when the body's core temperature lowers to_____.

   a. 98°F

   b. 95°F

   c. 90°F

   d. 85°F

   e. 80°F

7. A/n_____would cause a patient to present with lower back and right lower quadrant pain.

   a. aortic aneurysm

   b. kidney infection

   c. duodenal ulcer

   d. spleen contusion

   e. both a. and d.

8. Referred pain to the left shoulder due to a ruptured spleen is called_____.

   a. rebound pain

   b. Kehr's sign

   c. Braxton Hicks sign

   d. percussion pain

   e. axon-reflex sign

9. Traumatic injuries to the_____would cause the patient to present with uncoordinated and segmental robot-like movements.

   a. cerebrum

   b. cerebellum

   c. basal ganglia

   d. pons

   e. medulla oblongata

10. Which of the following would constitute a HIPAA violation?

   a. failure to provide patient with personal health information upon request

   b. unauthorized access of personal health information

   c. unauthorized sharing of personal health information on social media

   d. failure to enter HIPAA compliance agreement with vendors

   e. all of the above

11. _____is a condition caused by aspirin ingestion in children.

   a. Raynaud's disease

   b. Pyrexia

   c. Rheumatic fever

   d. Reye's syndrome

   e. RSV

12. Which of the following are parts of the running gait cycle that are most likely to produce a hamstring strain?

    Choose all that apply.

    a. early stance

    b. midstance

    c. late stance

    d. early swing

    e. late swing

13. A neurological issue causing the inability of the 5th finger to maintain adduction is called_____.

    a. clawhand position

    b. Volkmann's contracture

    c. radial tunnel syndrome

    d. Dupuytren's contracture

    e. Wartenberg sign

14. The_____runs at a 90 degree angle to the frontal plane.

    a. sagittal axis

    b. frontal axis

    c. horizontal axis

    d. all of the above

    e. both a. and c.

15. Which of the following is/are aspects of the female athlete triad?

    Choose all that apply.

    a. eating disorder

    b. depression

    c. menorrhagia

    d. pregnancy

    e. osteoporosis

    f. anemia

16. The critical core body temperature threshold for exertional heat stroke is_____.

    a. 100°F

    b. 103°F

    c. 105°F

    d. 108°F

    e. 110°F

17. The_____is a muscle that stabilizes the 12th rib during inspiration and laterally flexes the trunk to the same side.

    a. erector spinae

    b. rhomboids

    c. quadratus lumborum

    d. multifidus

    e. internal oblique

18. The concept of providing medical services within the legal bounds of professional training and expertise to avoid legal harm is called_____.

    a. guidelines

    b. practice standards

    c. scope of practice

    d. state practice act

    e. Hippocratic oath

19. An athlete is diagnosed with thoracic outlet syndrome and forward rounded shoulder posture is the primary contributing factor. Which of the following would be the most appropriate treatments?

    Choose all that apply.

    a. pectoralis major stretching

    b. rhomboids stretching

    c. strengthening exercises for the anterior neck musculature

    d. strengthening exercises for the scapulothoracic musculature

    e. cervical spine rotation strengthening

20. Which of the following are benefits to initiating closed kinetic chain exercises?

    Choose all that apply

    a. joint isolation

    b. proprioception

    c. joint stability

    d. muscle group isolation

    e. flexibility

21. An athlete is diagnosed with a radial nerve injury. Which of the following muscles would be affected?

Choose all that apply.

   a. biceps brachii

   b. anconeus

   c. deltoid

   d. brachioradialis

   e. pronator teres

22. _____are more common in skeletally mature individuals.

   a. Supracondylar fractures

   b. Olecranon fractures

23. The knee's lateral collateral ligament_____.

   a. has a proximal attachment to the joint capsule

   b. has a distal attachment on the lateral meniscus

   c. has a proximal attachment on the lateral femoral condyle

   d. protects the knee against valgus force

   e. all of the above

24. Anaerobic fitness can best be measured by using which of the following?

   a. VO$_2$ max testing

   b. plyometrics

   c. swimming

   d. treadmill walking

   e. upper body ergometer

25. _____ is a type of exercise in which resistance is applied by the clinician or therapist.

   a. Active resistance exercise

   b. Manual resistance exercise

   c. Dynamic resistance exercise

   d. Variable resistance exercise

   e. All of the above

26. This condition is characterized by a sudden and painless loss of vision. The loss of vision can be described as a "curtain falling across one's line of sight."

   a. hyphema

   b. globe rupture

   c. cataract

   d. retinal detachment

   e. astigmatism

27. Which of the following are contraindications to resistance exercise?
   Choose all that apply.

   a. inflammation

   b. obesity

   c. type-1 diabetes

   d. type-2 diabetes

   e. carditis

   f. congestive heart failure

   g. pregnancy

28. _____refers to the deformation of tissue over time.

   a. Mechanical stress

   b. Tissue load

   c. Strain

   d. Stress

   e. Creep

29. _____is a pair of ligaments that connect the lamina of one vertebra to the vertebrae above.

   a. Ligamentum nuchae

   b. Ligamentum flavum

   c. Supraspinous ligament

   d. Interspinous ligament

   e. Posterior interspinous ligament

30. _____is a diagnostic tool for detecting dural irritation and facet joint compression.

   a. Slump test

   b. Straight leg raise test

   c. Well straight leg raise test

   d. Quadrant test

   e. All of the above

31. The area between the superior and middle glenohumeral ligaments is called the_____ and is a weak spot in the glenohumeral joint capsule.

   a. inferior pouch

   b. foramen of Weitbrecht

   c. coracoacromial arch

   d. coracohumeral ligament

   e. glenoid cavity

32. The_____is a structure formed by the pisiform and hook of hamate, and the ulnar nerve passes through it.

    a. tunnel of Guyon

    b. carpal tunnel

    c. arcade of Struthers

    d. foramen of Weitbrecht

    e. foramen of Winslow

33. An injury to the left and right pars interarticularis with associated spinal instability is known as a/n_____.

    a. spondylolysis

    b. spondylolisthesis

    c. hangman's fracture

    d. ring fracture

    e. Jefferson fracture

34. _____rank(s) as second to cardiac-related injuries and illnesses as the most common

    cause of death in football.

    a. Shock

    b. Catastrophic brain injuries

    c. Respiratory emergencies

    d. Heat illnesses

    e. Cervical spine injuries

35. Which of the following are symptoms of hyperglycemia?

    Choose all that apply.

    a. nervousness

    b. nausea

    c. fatigue

    d. thirst

    e. loss of consciousness

    f. dizziness

    g. trembling

36. The active compression test (O'Brien test) is used to identify_____.

    a. sternoclavicular injury

    b. rotator cuff tendinopathy

    c. SLAP lesion

    d. thoracic outlet syndrome

    e. posterior glenohumeral instability

37. A baseball player is batting. He is struck in the chest by a fast ball and immediately collapses. He is not breathing and has no pulse. What condition do you suspect and what is the next most appropriate step?

    a.. Myocardial infarction; get him to cath lab right away

    b. Aortic dissection; give him mouth to mouth and call EMS

    c. Commotio cordis; activate EMS, start immediate CPR and get AED

    d. Myocarditis; start immediate CPR and get AED

    e. Hypoglycemia; Give him 15-20 g of oral glucose-containing solution and reassess

38. NSAIDs work by what mechanism?

    a. inhibit COX1/COX2 in the inflammatory pathway

    b. block platelet production

    c. inhibit arachidonic acid production

    d. target pain receptors in the brain but do not affect inflammation

39. Which of the following are signs/symptoms of hypovolemic shock?

    Choose all that apply.

    a. increased blood pressure

    b. decreased blood pressure

    c. excessive thirst

    d. cyanosis

    e. slow pulse

    f. strong pulse

    g. red skin

40. _____consist(s) of a quick moving eccentric activity followed by a burst of concentric activity.

    a. Isometrics

    b. Isotonics

    c. Isokinetics

    d. Plyometrics

    e. Sports specific activities

41. Which of the following are components of the feedforward mechanism?

   Choose all that apply.

   a. preparatory muscle activity

   b. real time planning based on past experiences

   c. reflexive muscular activity

   d. reactive muscular activity

   e. unplanned muscular activity

42. Which mechanoreceptor is responsible for detecting skin stretching?

   a. hair follicles

   b. Meissner corpuscles

   c. Pacinian corpuscles

   d. Merkel cells

   e. Ruffini corpuscles

43. The_____is a heart structure that contracts and delivers blood into the pulmonary artery.

   a. right atrium

   b. left atrium

   c. right ventricle

   d. left ventricle

   e. aorta

44. A/n_____is a pathology to the superior labrum.

   a. SLAP lesion

   b. Bankart lesion

   c. Hill-Sachs lesion

   d. Stener lesion

   e. reverse Bankart lesion

45. Which of the following electrical stimulation techniques identifies the characteristics listed below?

   Intensity: Enough to produce 60% of max isometric contraction

   Pulses per second: 70-85

   Cycle: 10-15 seconds on and 1 minute off

   a. premodulated current

   b. interferential current

   c. high volt pulsed biphasic

   d. low volt Russian current

   e. high volt Russian current

46. Which of the following are components of General Adaptation Syndrome?

   Choose all that apply.

   a. adaptation

   b. alarm

   c. resistance

   d. reeducation

   e. emotion

   f. elasticity

   g. exhaustion

47. All nociceptive and thermal neural signals travel on_____pathways.

    a. A-delta

    b. B-alpha

    c. C

    d. both a. and c.

    e. all of the above

48. An athlete is diagnosed with a Grade 2 MCL sprain that occurred 2 days ago. Which of the following would

    be priorities for treatment of this injury during this time?

    Choose all that apply.

    a. inflammation control

    b. pain control

    c. sports-specific activities

    d. range of motion

    e. isotonic exercises

    f. isokinetic exercises

    g. proprioception

49. Which grade of Maitland's Scale of Joint Mobilizations is a small amplitude thrust at the end range of motion

    that bumps into the restriction?

    a. Grade 1

    b. Grade 2

    c. Grade 3

    d. Grade 4

    e. Grade 5

50. Which of the following diagnostic special tests is used to demonstrate carpal tunnel syndrome?

    a. Hawkins-Kennedy test

    b. Roos test

    c. Phalen's test

    d. Bunnell-Littler test

    e. Froment's sign

51. Dehydration is characterized by a minimum of_____loss in body weight.

    a. 1-2%

    b. 3-5%

    c. 5-7%

    d. 7-10%

    e. 10-15%

52. What is the loose-packed position of the hip called?

    a. tailor's position

    b. Legg-Calve-Perthes position

    c. Bonnet position

    d. FABER position

    e. anatomical position

53._____is a budget where all items must be justified with no regard to previous spending behaviors or patterns. Budgeting categories and items are ranked in order of importance.

a. Line-item

b. Zero-based

c. Spending-ceiling

d. Open

e. program

54. Which of the following are return-to-play criteria for an athlete diagnosed with a viral skin infection?

Choose all that apply.

a. 72 hour minimum of antiviral treatment

b. 120 hour minimum of antiviral treatment

c. no fever

d. draining lesions

e. no new blisters for 24 hours

f. no new blisters for 72 hours

g. firm crust on lesions

h. malaise

i. sleep disturbance

j. new blister formation

55. Which of the following are intrinsic factors of overuse injuries?

   Choose all that apply.

   a. height

   b. environment

   c. recovery

   d. training

   e. technique

   f. Tanner stage

   g. conditioning

   h. laxity

Matching Section (Simulates Drag and Drop Questions)

Match the terms on the left with their corresponding description.

Topic: Acute Skin Trauma

56._____antiseptic   a. flush wound

57._____debridement   b. foam dressing

58._____Polymem   c. sodium hypochlorite

59._____Dermabond   d. remove wound debris

60._____irrigation   e. wound adhesive

61. Which of the following are contraindications to aquatic therapy?

   Choose all that apply.

   a. fear of water

   b. obesity

   c. sinusitis

   d. open wounds

   e. sunburn

62. _____occurs when the patient experiences severe and sometimes sudden abdominal pain due to inflammation of the peritoneum.

   a. Appendicitis

   b. Pancreatitis

   c. Acute cholecystitis

   d. Colic

   e. Acute abdomen

63. The arrow in the picture below is pointing to which structure?

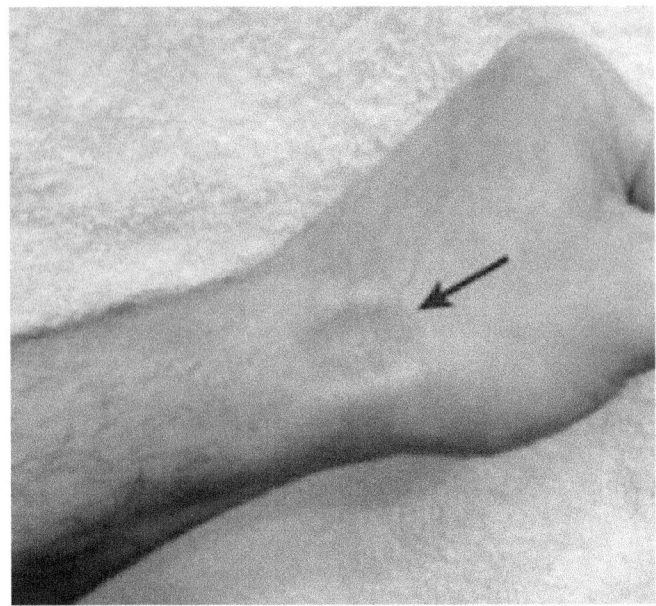

    a. anatomical snuff box

    b. hypothenar eminence

    c. TFCC

    d. thenar eminence

    e. radial head

64. _____is a bilateral pars interarticularis fracture of C2 with an associated dislocation of C2-C3.

    a. Jefferson fracture

    b. Hangman's fracture

    c. Wedge fracture

    d. Spondylolysis

    e. Spondylolisthesis

65._____allows an individual to pursue opportunities of interest and the ability to achieve

life balance through those opportunities.

a. Social wellness

b. Emotional wellness

c. Spiritual wellness

d. Environmental wellness

e. Occupational wellness

66. _____is the pain control technique that utilizes A-beta fibers in order to block sensations from using second

order neurons.

a. Gate control

b. Endogenous opiates

c. Central-biasing

d. Visualization

e. Neurotransmitter centering

67. How should a concussed athlete be notified of the instructions for home care of his or her injury?

a. verbally

b. written or printed

c. email

d. both a. and b.

e. all of the above

68. The goal for treating an exertional heat stroke victim is to_____within 30 minutes after collapse.

    a. lower body temperature below 102°F

    b. lower body temperature below 96°F

    c. administer 1 L of fluids

    d. administer supplemental oxygen gas

    e. return to play

69. _____is required in order to treat a conscious and mentally competent adult before care is initiated.

    a. Cause

    b. Duty

    c. Consent

    d. Standards of practice

    e. All of the above

70. Most cases of_____occur when endurance athletes ingest excessive amounts of hypotonic liquid.

    a. dehydration

    b. exertional hyponatremia

    c. exertional rhabdomyolysis

    d. exertional sickling

    e. hypoglycemia

71. Which of the following are environmental risks for cancer?

   Choose all that apply.

   a. smoking

   b. obesity

   c. genetics

   d. air pollution

   e. ultraviolet rays

72. What is true of fitting a tennis racquet?

   a. A heavy racquet requires less strength.

   b. Stiff or tightly wound strings place more stress on the wrist and hand.

   c. Loose wound strings place more stress on the wrist and hand.

   d. A large grip adds more stress to the wrist and hand.

   e. A small grip adds less stress to the wrist and hand.

73. What is the most comfortable and advised position for an athlete following a grade-1 acromioclavicular

   sprain?

   a. anatomical position

   b. braced position

   c. tailor's position

   d. neutral shoulder position

   e. protracted position

74. An athlete with a positive sulcus and Feagan test likely has_____.

   a. anterior glenohumeral instability

   b. inferior glenohumeral instability

   c. posterior glenohumeral instability

   d. thoracic outlet syndrome

   e. multidirectional glenohumeral instability

75. An athlete with shoulder impingement is likely to have_____.

   a. subtendinous bursitis

   b. gross internal rotation deficit

   c. rotator cuff tendinopathy

   d. bicipital tendonitis

   e. all of the above

76. Which of the following are effects of joint immobilization following an injury?

   Choose all that apply.

   a. increased collagen cross-links

   b. decreased collagen cross-links

   c. fiber meshwork contracts

   d. reduced range of motion

   e. increased range of motion

   f. increased blood flow to area

77. _____is used to assess visual acuity during a pre-participation evaluation.

   a. Snellen chart

   b. Ishihara test

   c. Zeiss test

   d. Visual field test

   e. PERRLA

78. Which of the following antibiotics are bacteriostatic?

   a. sulfa

   b. penicillin

   c. keflex

   d. cephalosporins

   e. all of the above

79. The risk of soft tissue injury during pregnancy increases due to the body's production of _____.

   a. human chorionic gonadotropin

   b. estrogen

   c. relaxin

   d. oxytocin

   e. progesterone

80. Which of the following are treatments for heat exhaustion?

Choose all that apply.

a. tighten clothing

b. initiate oxygen gas supplementation

c. apply hydrocollator packs to armpits and neck

d. return to play within 15 minutes

e. place in shock position

End of Exam 4

Exam 4 Answers

1. b. III
2. b. III
3. a. d. e. II
4. b. IV
5. a. I
6. b. I
7. a. III
8. b. III
9. b. III
10. e. V
11. d. IV
12. c. e. II
13. e. II
14. a. I
15. a. e. I
16. c. III
17. c. I
18. c. V
19. a. d. IV
20. b. c. IV
21. b. d. II
22. b. II
23. c. I
24. b. I
25. b. IV
26. d. II
27. a. e. f. IV
28. e. I
29. b. I
30. d. II
31. b. II
32. a. I
33. b. II
34. b. III
35. b. c. d. II
36. c. II
37. c. III
38. a. IV
39. b. c. d. III
40. d. IV

41. a. b. IV
42. e. I
43. c. I
44. a. II
45. e. IV
46. b. c. g. I
47. d. I
48. a. b. IV
49. d. IV
50. c. II
51. b. I
52. c. I
53. b. V
54. b. c. f. g. IV
55. a. f. h. II
56. c. IV
57. d. IV
58. b. IV
59. e. IV
60. a. IV
61. a. d. IV
62. e. III
63. a. I
64. b. III
65. e. I
66. a. IV
67. d. II
68. a. III
69. c. V
70. b. I
71. d. e. I
72. b. I
73. b. IV
74. d. II
75. b. II
76. a. c. d. IV
77. a. I
78. a. IV
79. c. I
80. b. e. III

Exam 5 on next page

Exam 5

80 Questions

4 hour maximum

1. Which of the following would contribute to an increased risk of heatstroke?

    a. caffeine

    b. alcohol

    c. diarrhea

    d. sickle-cell trait

    e. all of the above

2. Which of the following heat illnesses is characterized by skin that is red and dry?

    a. heat cramps

    b. heat exhaustion

    c. heat stroke

    d. heat syncope

    e. all of the above

3. Preiser's disease is described as idiopathic avascular necrosis of what bone?

    a. femur

    b. clavicle

    c. scaphoid

    d. cuboid

    e. lunate

4. In young individuals, a traction force combined with pronation of the forearm can result in a radioulnar joint dislocation, commonly known as a/n_____.

   a. milkmaid's sign

   b. terrible triad of the elbow

   c. nursemaid's elbow

   d. little league elbow

   e. cubital tunnel syndrome

5. The deltoid is innervated by the_____nerve.

   a. axillary

   b. radial

   c. ulnar

   d. spinal accessory

   e. median

6. Which of the following is a diagnostic test for DeQuervain's syndrome?

   a. Watson test

   b. Phalen's test

   c. Bunnell-Littler test

   d. Froment's sign

   e. Finkelstein's test

7. The duty cycle when using phonophoresis should be_____.

   a. 20%

   b. 40%

   c. 50%

   d. 75%

   e. 100%

8. The technical term for joint accessory motion is_____.

    a. osteokinematic

    b. arthrokinematic

    c. passive motion

    d. active motion

    e. complex motion

9. High-pulse frequency, short phase duration and sensory level currents of electrical stimulation invoke the_____of pain modulation.

    a. enkephalin mechanism

    b. endogenous opiates

    c. gate mechanism

    d. descending pathways

    e. all of the above

10. _____is the most appropriate diagnostic test for hip flexor tightness.

    a. Homan's sign

    b. Thompson test

    c. Thomas test

    d. Patrick's test

    e. Hip scouring test

11. An adult's resting heart rate is measured at 90 beats per minute. What is the classification of this heart rate?

   a. normal

   b. tachycardia

   c. bradycardia

12. An adult's breathing rate of 8 breaths per minute is classified as what?

   a. normal

   b. bradypnea

   c. tachypnea

   d. dyspnea

13. Which of the following is a special test for PCL injury?

   a. lateral pivot shift test

   b. Slocum test for anteromedial rotary instability

   c. Hughston's test

   d. sweep test

   e. quadriceps active test

14. The dose of epinephrine in an adult EpiPen® is_____.

   a. 0.15 mg

   b. 0.3 mg

   c. 0.5 mg

   d. 1 mg

   e. 1.5 mg

15. _____are mechanical, thermal, or chemical pain receptors in tissue.

    a. Merkel's discs

    b. Meissner's corpuscles

    c. Pacinian corpuscles

    d. Ruffini corpuscles

    e. Nociceptors

16. Which of the following is the appropriate exercise progression during the rehabilitation process?

    a. isometric-isotonic-isokinetic-plyometric

    b. isotonic-isokinetic-isometric-plyometric

    c. isotonic-isometric-isokinetic-plyometric

    d. isometric-isokinetic-isotonic-plyometric

    e. isometric-isotonic-plyometric-isokinetic

17. _____is a type of budget where there is no set budget but purchasing or spending on each and every item must be justified for its cost and need.

    a. Lump-sum

    b. Line-item

    c. Fixed

    d. Zero-based

    e. Spending-ceiling model

18. Which of the following are signs and/or symptoms of dehydration?

Choose all that apply.

a. cramps

b. bradycardia

c. decreased core body temperature

d. alertness

e. decreased athletic performance

19. Which of the following are classified as B vitamins?

Choose all that apply.

a. niacin

b. folate

c. iodine

d. fluorine

e. pantothenic acid

f. phosphorus

g. ascorbic acid

20. Which of the following are some deconditioning effects of an athlete undergoing bed rest for a prolonged period of time?

Choose all that apply.

a. decreased exercise tolerance

b. decreased plasma volume

c. decreased bone mineral density

d. increased mitochondrial concentration

e. increased stroke volume

f. increased muscular strength

g. increased VO_{2max}

21. A_____is a measure representing the amount of heat energy necessary to raise 1kg of water 1°C.

   a. kilojoule

   b. kilowatt

   c. kilocalorie

   d. kiloMET

   e. kilokelvin

22. The_____of exercise is the product of frequency, intensity, and duration.

   a. volume

   b. load

   c. periodization

   d. overload

   e. all of the above

23. During which phase of healing does fibronectin bind fibrin and collagen to form a barrier in order to stop bleeding?

   a. inflammation

   b. proliferation

   c. maturation

24. A Certified Athletic Trainer fails to follow up on a symptomatic athlete with a concussion. This failure results in permanent brain damage. It is later determined that a reasonable Certified Athletic Trainer should have performed this duty. This is an example of_____.

   a. misfeasance

   b. malfeasance

   c. nonfeasance

   d. all of the above

25. A 38 year old male professional golfer presents with pain that radiates from his neck into the left trapezius, scapula, shoulder, arm, wrist, and hand. These symptoms increase and include paresthesia in the same areas as the day progresses. Based on the history, which pathology would you suspect?

a. brachial plexus trauma

b. cervical nerve root compression

c. thoracic outlet syndrome

d. clinical cervical instability

e. cervical stenosis

26. In the diagram below, draw a small circle in the area of the **gallbladder**.

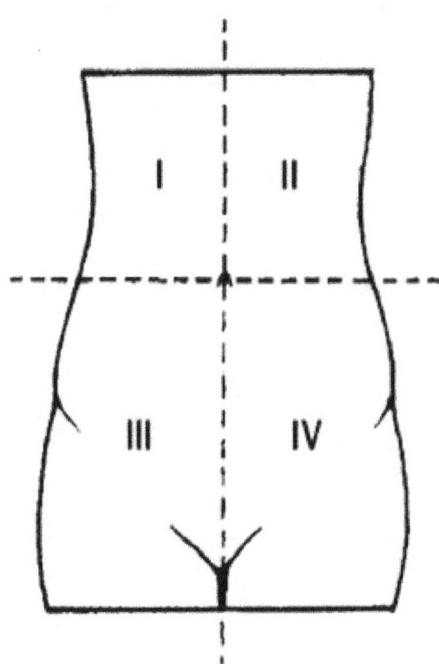

27. Tightness of what structure causes an exaggerated anterior pelvic tilt and lumbar lordosis?

    a. hamstrings

    b. rectus abdominis

    c. piriformis

    d. hip flexors

    e. gluteus maximus

28. Which of the following diagnostic tests is used to identify IT band tightness?

    a. Thomas test

    b. Ober's test

    c. FABER test

    d. quadrant test

    e. Both b. and d.

29. The normal respiration rate range for a young adult is_____.

    a. 10-12 breaths per minute

    b. 12-15 breaths per minute

    c. 15-18 breaths per minute

    d. 18-23 breaths per minute

    e. 25-30 breaths per minute

30. The_____is the perimeter of the contact area between the body and the support surface that it is in contact with.

    a. center of mass

    b. center of gravity

    c. center of pressure

    d. base of support

    e. all of the above

31. _____are legal wrongs committed against the person or property of another.

    a. Torts

    b. Negligence

    c. Misfeasance

    d. Malfeasance

    e. Nonfeasance

32. Which of the following would be most likely to sustain a spondylolysis based on the information provided?

    a. youth swimmer

    b. adolescent gymnast

    c. teen football player

    d. adult tennis player

    e. elderly cyclist

33. Which of the following is a fungal infection of the skin in the groin region?

    a. tinea cruris

    b. tinea pedis

    c. tinea capitis

    d. candidiasis

    e. pyoderma

34. What is the medical term for an infection of a fingernail's bed?

    a. felon

    b. subungual hematoma

    c. paronychia

    d. ganglion cyst

    e. hordeolum

35. Monophasic electrical stimulation current is used for_____.

    a. pain modulation

    b. muscle contraction

    c. movement of ions

    d. all of the above

36. _____are high-threshold tissue receptors that sense mechanical pressure.

    a. Merkel's discs

    b. Meissner's corpuscles

    c. Pacinian corpuscles

    d. Ruffini corpuscles

    e. Nociceptors

37. Which of the following muscles provide external rotation of the glenohumeral joint?

    Choose all that apply.

    a. infraspinatus

    b. subscapularis

    c. teres minor

    d. supraspinatus

    e. teres major

    f. coracobrachialis

38. _____is a rheumatic condition that first appears during adolescence and is characterized by the ossification of the anterior and posterior longitudinal spinal ligaments and facet joints.

    a. Scheuermann's disease

    b. ankylosing spondylitis

    c. Rickets

    d. Osteosarcoma

    e. Huntington's disease

39. _____is a congenital condition involving one or both scapulae being undescended.

   a. Scapular dyskinesis

   b. Sprengel's deformity

   c. Step deformity

   d. Russell's sign

   e. Thoracic outlet syndrome

40. Which of the following provides knee posterolateral rotatory stability?

   a. anterior cruciate ligament

   b. posterior cruciate ligament

   c. arcuate ligament

   d. medial collateral ligament

   e. all of the above

41. _____is a clinical evaluation method used to detect osteochondral defects.

   a. Wilson's test

   b. Ober's test

   c. McMurray's test

   d. Apley's compression test

   e. All of the above

42. The PROP acronym for shock treatment stands for_____.

   a. position, rest, oxygen, positive reinforcement

   b. positive reinforcement, rest, oxygen, position

   c. position, reassure, oxygen, positive pressure ventilation

   d. position, reassure, oxygen, reposition

   e. Position, rest, oxygen, reposition

43. The amount of time that it takes to transition from an eccentric to concentric contraction is called_____.

    a. temporal contraction
    b. amortization
    c. cocking
    d. series elastic timing
    e. angular transitioning

44. Which of the following are characteristics of the feedback mechanism?
    Choose all that apply.
    a. preparatory muscular activity
    b. planned movements based on patterns from past experience
    c. reflexive muscular activity
    d. reactive muscular activity
    e. anticipatory muscular activity

45. The ability to control the movement of the body or body segment during rapid movement is known as_____.

    a. agility
    b. coordination
    c. power
    d. stability
    e. balance

46._____refers to the adequate circulation of blood within a tissue in order to supply its oxygen demand.

    a. Amortization
    b. Perfusion
    c. Stroke volume
    d. VO$_2$ max
    e. Critical need

47. A collegiate female soccer player gets hit on the face with a ball during play. The athlete presents with bleeding from the nose. The medical term for this condition is_____.

    a. epistaxis

    b. hemotympanum

    c. otopyorrhea

    d. ecchymosis

    e. edema

48. Which of the following is a characteristic of capillary bleeding?

    a. oozing

    b. squirting

    c. dark blood

    d. pulsing

    e. nonstop

49. _____is the medical term for vomiting blood.

    a. Hematuria

    b. Hematemesis

    c. Hematochezia

    d. Hemotympanum

    e. Otopyorrhea

50. The adaptation of bone tissue to submaximal stressors over time is known as_____.

    a. SAID principle

    b. Wolff's law

    c. Hooke's law

    d. Davis's law

    e. All of the above

51. _____is an ischemic condition of the femoral head that usually occurs during the first decade of life and causes decreased hip abduction and internal rotation.

    a. Slipped capital femoral epiphysis syndrome

    b. CAM lesion

    c. Pincer lesion

    d. Legg-Calve-Perthes disease

    e. Osteitis pubis

52. What is the return-to-play criteria for an athlete with a skin fungal infection?

    Choose all that apply.

    a. topical fungicide for at least 72 hours

    b. topical fungicide for at least one week

    c. non-permeable membrane dressing

    d. liquid-permeable membrane dressing

    e. gas-permeable membrane dressing

53. Which of the following are methods by which thermal energy is lost in the human body?

    Choose all that apply.

    a. radiation

    b. cavitation

    c. entropy

    d. evaporation

    e. photogenesis

54. _____is a pattern characterized by alternating between deep and slow or absent breathing.

   a. Eupnea

   b. Kussmaul breathing

   c. Cheyne-Stokes respirations

   d. Apneustic breathing

   e. Biot's breathing

55. Which of the following would be an effective medication for treating irritable bowel syndrome?

   a. loperamide (Imodium)

   b. ibuprofen (Motrin)

   c. acetaminophen (Tylenol)

   d. naproxen sodium (Aleve)

   e. topical starch (Tucks)

56. Which of the following is/are true regarding dietary supplements?

   Choose all that apply.

   a. They are regulated by the FDA.

   b. Evidence of safety is required.

   c. Athletic Trainers should be prepared to educate athletes on supplements.

   d. Athletic Trainers should employ a food-first philosophy regarding supplements.

   e. Multivitamins are required to be tested for purity.

57. What is true regarding overuse injuries in pediatric athletics?

Choose all that apply.

a. Coaches and parents should be educated in this topic.

b. Injury surveillance and recording is not important because of age changes.

c. Pre Participation Examinations are a vital part of overuse injury prevention in this demographic.

d. Rules and guidelines cannot be modified in order to prevent overuse injuries in this demographic.

e. The amount of repetitive sport activity can be limited in order to prevent overuse injuries in this demographic.

Matching Section (Simulates Drag and Drop)

Match the term on the left with its corresponding description on the right.

Questions 58-61

Topic: Intracranial Pathologies

58._____concussion   a. leading athletic cause of death within 24 hours of injury

59._____subdural hematoma   b. mild traumatic brain injury

60._____subarachnoid hemorrhage   c. creates "star of death"

61._____epidural hematoma   d. lucid interval after injury

62. Which of the following shoulder motions are components of D2 Extension PNF patterns of movement?

Choose all that apply.

a. extension

b. flexion

c. abduction

d. external rotation

e. adduction

f. internal rotation

63. _____ is a virus that causes mononucleosis.

    a. retrovirus

    b. norovirus

    c. varicella zoster virus

    d. Epstein-Barr virus

    e. parvovirus

64. Which of the following would best describe the location of the frontal cranial bone as it relates to the whole human body?

    a. anterior, medial, inferior

    b. lateral, superior, anterior, medial, posterior

    c anterior, lateral, superior

    d. anterior, medial, superior

    e. posterior, medial, superior

65. Tenderness in the_____ is indicative of kidney pathology.

    a. angle of Louis

    b. costovertebral angle

    c. costal arch

    d. sternal angle

    e. jugular notch

66. Point tenderness beneath the structure the arrow is pointing at is indicative of what injury?

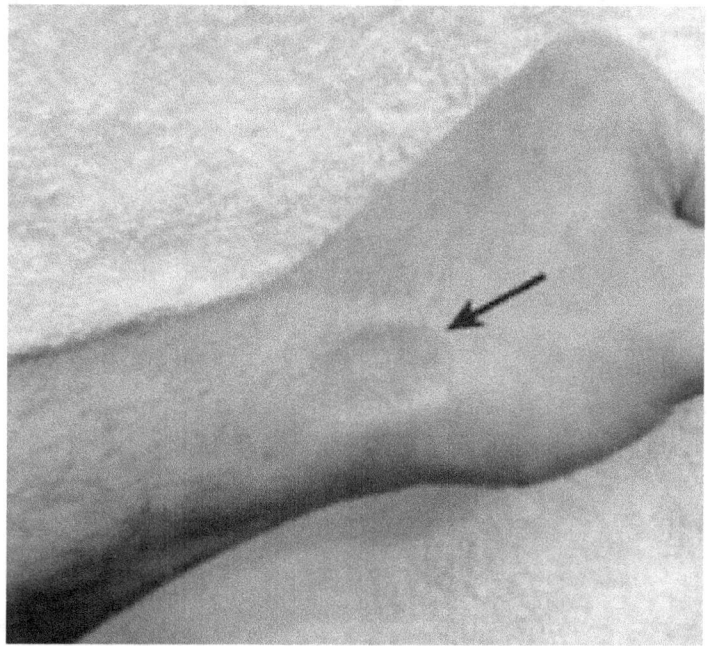

a. capitate injury

b. scaphoid injury

c. lunate injury

d. radial injury

e. TFCC injury

67. Nursemaid's elbow is an injury that involves disruption of what structure?

a. RCL

b. UCL

c. annular ligament

d. TFCC

e. radial notch

68. A positive halo test indicates an injury that causes_____.

  a. intracranial bleeding

  b. cerebrospinal fluid leakage

  c. second impact syndrome

  d. dehydration

  e. rhabdomyolysis

69. _____is caused by hemisection of the spinothalamic tracts of the spinal cord and causes ipsilateral motor

weakness and contralateral sensation deficits.

  a. Brown-Sequard syndrome

  b. Tetraplegia

  c. Central cord syndrome

  d. Anterior cord syndrome

  e. Transverse myelitis

70. _____is an inherited cardiac condition characterized by an arrhythmia that prolongs repolarization.

  a. Atrial flutter

  b. Atrial fibrillation

  c. Ventricular fibrillation

  d. Long QT syndrome

  e. Paroxysmal arrhythmia

71. Articular cartilage is composed of_____and has a long healing process.

  a. type I collagen

  b. type II collagen

  c. type III collagen

  d. elastin

  e. bony callus

72. Which of the following is a diagnostic assessment of postural stability?

   a. BESS

   b. AVPU

   c. GCS

   d. TUG

   e. All of the above

73. _____is the ability to handle stress and changes in life's circumstances.

   a. Social wellness

   b. Emotional wellness

   c. Spiritual wellness

   d. Environmental wellness

   e. Intellectual wellness

74. Which of the following are treatments of an athlete experiencing exertional sickling?

   Choose all that apply.

   a. immediate withdrawal from activity

   b. cryotherapy

   c. thermal modalities

   d. administer oxygen

   e. monitor vitals

75. When play is postponed due to lightning, it shall not be resumed until lightning or thunder is absent for a period of_____.

   a. 10 minutes

   b. 15 minutes

   c. 30 minutes

   d. 45 minutes

   e. 60 minutes

76._____should be suspected if an athlete experiences a sudden collapse and is unresponsive.

   a. Seizure

   b. Shock

   c. Sudden cardiac arrest

   d. Stroke

   e. Exertional sickling

77._____occurs when prolonged exposure to cold and wet environments causes small erythematous papules, edema, itching and pain to occur.

   a. Frostnip

   b. Frostbite

   c. Hypothermia

   d. Immersion foot

   e. Chillblains

78. Which of the following should be considered when deciding on whether to remove equipment from an athlete during an emergency?

   Choose all that apply.

   a. expenses

   b. access to airway

   c. alignment of cervical spine

   d. comfort

   e. bleeding

79. A geriatric tennis player presents with shoulder pain that has progressed over the past month. The patient has weakness associated with internal rotation and adduction of the shoulder. What is your initial assessment based on the information provided?

   a. supraspinatus tendinopathy

   b. subscapularis tendinopathy

   c. teres minor tendinopathy

   d. infraspinatus tendinopathy

   e. impingement

80. Which of the following are lower extremity plyometric exercises for ACL injury prevention?

  Choose all that apply.

   a. tuck jump

   b. high knee skipping

   c. zigzag shuffle

   d. squat jump

   e. shuttle run

End of Exam 5

Exam 5 Answers/Domains

1. e. I
2. c. I
3. c. II
4. c. II
5. a. I
6. e. II
7. e. IV
8. b. I
9. c. IV
10. c. II
11. a. I
12. b. I
13. e. II
14. b. III
15. e. I
16. a. IV
17. d. V
18. a. e. I
19. a. b. e. I
20. a. b. c. I
21. c. I
22. a. I
23. a. IV
24. c. V
25. c. II
26. upper right quadrant. I
27. d. II
28. b. II
29. b. I
30. d. I
31. a. V
32. b. II
33. a. II
34. c. II
35. d. IV
36. c. I
37. a. c. I
38. b. II
39. b. II
40. d. I

41. a. II
42. c. III
43. b. I
44. c. d. IV
45. a. I
46. b. I
47. a. II
48. a. II
49. b. II
50. b. I
51. d. II
52. a. e. IV
53. a. d. I
54. c. III
55. a. IV
56. c. d. V
57. a. e. I
58. b. III
59. a. III
60. c. III
61. d. III
62. a. f. e. IV
63. d. I
64. d. I
65. b. III
66. b. II
67. c. II
68. b. III
69. a. III
70. d. I
71. b. IV
72. a. I
73. b. I
74. a. d. e. III
75. c. I
76. c. III
77. e. I
78. b. c. e. III
79. b. II
80. a. d. IV

Bibliography

Beam, J. W., Buckley, B., Holcomb, W. R., & Ciocca, M. (2016). National Athletic Trainers' Association position statement: Management of Acute Skin Trauma. *Journal of Athletic Training, 51*(12), 1053–1070. https://doi.org/10.4085/1062-6050-51.7.01

Biel, A., & Dorn, R. (2019). *Trail Guide to the body: A hands-on guide to locating muscles, bones and more (6th ed.)* (6th ed.). Books of Discovery.

Bonci, C. M., Bonci, L. J., Granger, L. R., Johnson, C. L., Malina, R. M., Milne, L. W., Ryan, R. R., & Vanderbunt, E. M. (2008). National Athletic Trainers' Association position statement: Preventing, detecting, and managing disordered eating in athletes. *Journal of Athletic Training, 43*(1), 80–108. https://doi.org/10.4085/1062-6050-43.1.80

Broglio, S. P., Cantu, R. C., Gioia, G. A., Guskiewicz, K. M., Kutcher, J., Palm, M., & McLeod, T. C. (2014). National Athletic Trainers' Association position statement: Management of Sport Concussion. *Journal of Athletic Training, 49*(2), 245–265. https://doi.org/10.4085/1062-6050-49.1.07

Cappaert, T. A., Stone, J. A., Castellani, J. W., Krause, B. A., Smith, D., & Stephens, B. A. (2008). National Athletic Trainers' Association position statement: Environmental cold injuries. *Journal of Athletic Training, 43*(6), 640–658. https://doi.org/10.4085/1062-6050-43.6.640

Casa, D. J., DeMartini, J. K., Bergeron, M. F., Csillan, D., Eichner, E. R., Lopez, R. M., Ferrara, M. S., Miller, K. C., O'Connor, F., Sawka, M. N., & Yeargin, S. W. (2015). National Athletic Trainers' Association position statement: Exertional Heat illnesses. *Journal of Athletic Training.* https://doi.org/10.4085/1062-6050-50-9-07

Conley, K. M., Bolin, D. J., Carek, P. J., Konin, J. G., Neal, T. L., & Violette, D. (2014). National Athletic Trainers' Association position statement: Preparticipation physical examinations and disqualifying conditions. *Journal of Athletic Training, 49*(1), 102–120. https://doi.org/10.4085/1062-6050-48.6.05

Cuppett, M., & Walsh, K. M. (2012). *General medical conditions in the athlete.* Elsevier Mosby.

Donatelle, R. J. (2020). *Access to health.* Pearson Education, Inc.

Floyd, R. T. (2018). *Manual of Structural Kinesiology.* McGraw-Hill.

Gould, T. E., Piland, S. G., Caswell, S. V., Ranalli, D., Mills, S., Ferrara, M. S., & Courson, R. (2016). National Athletic Trainers' Association position statement: Preventing and managing sport-related dental and oral injuries. *Journal of Athletic Training, 51*(10), 821–839. https://doi.org/10.4085/1062-6050-51.8.01

H., M. R. M., Abrahams, P., Boon, J., & Spratt, J. (2008). *McMinn's clinical atlas of human anatomy*. Mosby Elsevier.

Houglum, J. E., Harrelson, G. L., & Seefeldt, T. M. (2016). *Principles of pharmacology for athletic trainers 3rd. Ed.* (3rd ed.). SLACK Incorporated.

Kisner, C., Colby, L. A., & Borstad, J. (2018). *Therapeutic exercise: Foundations and techniques* (7th ed.). F.A. Davis Company.

Krebs, C., Weinberg, J., Akesson, E. J., & Dilli, E. (2018). *Neuroscience*. Wolters Kluwer Health.

Masaracchio, M., & Frommer, C. (2014). *Clinical guide to musculoskeletal palpation*. Human Kinetics.

McDermott, B. P., Anderson, S. A., Armstrong, L. E., Casa, D. J., Cheuvront, S. N., Cooper, L., Kenney, W. L., O'Connor, F. G., & Roberts, W. O. (2017). National Athletic Trainers' Association position statement: Fluid Replacement for the physically active. *Journal of Athletic Training, 52*(9), 877–895. https://doi.org/10.4085/1062-6050-52.9.02

MCGINNIS, P. (2020). *Biomechanics of Sport and exercise* (4th ed.). HUMAN KINETICS.

Netter, F. H. (2019). *Atlas of human anatomy* (2nd ed.). Elsevier.

Padua, D. A., DiStefano, L. J., Hewett, T. E., Garrett, W. E., Marshall, S. W., Golden, G. M., Shultz, S. J., & Sigward, S. M. (2018). National Athletic Trainers' Association position statement: Prevention of Anterior Cruciate Ligament Injury. *Journal of Athletic Training, 53*(1), 5–19. https://doi.org/10.4085/1062-6050-99-16

Pfeiffer, R. P., Mangus, B. C., & Trowbridge, C. A. (2015). *Concepts of athletic training* (7th ed.). Jones &. Barlett Publ.

Prentice, W. E. (2021). *Principles of athletic training: A guide to evidence-based clinical practice* (17th ed.). McGraw-Hill.

Shultz, S. J., Houglum, P. A., & Perrin, D. H. (2016). *Examination of musculoskeletal injuries*. Human Kinetics.

Stanfield, C. L. (2017). *Principles of human physiology*. Pearson.

Starkey, C., & Brown, S. D. (2015). *Examination of Orthopedic & Athletic Injuries* (4th ed.). F.A. Davis Company.

Swartz, E. E., Boden, B. P., Courson, R. W., Decoster, L. C., Horodyski, M. B., Norkus, S. A., Rehberg, R. S., & Waninger, K. N. (2009). National Athletic Trainers' Association position statement: Acute management of the cervical spine–injured athlete. *Journal of Athletic Training, 44*(3), 306–331. https://doi.org/10.4085/1062-6050-44.3.306

Walsh, K. M., Cooper, M. A., Holle, R., Rakov, V. A., Roeder, W. P., & Ryan, M. (2013). National Athletic Trainers' Association position statement: Lightning safety for athletics and recreation. *Journal of Athletic Training, 48*(2), 258–270. https://doi.org/10.4085/1062-6050-48.2.25

Zinder, S. M., Basler, R. S., Foley, J., Scarlata, C., & Vasily, D. B. (2010). National Athletic Trainers' Association position statement: Skin diseases. *Journal of Athletic Training, 45*(4), 411–428. https://doi.org/10.4085/1062-6050-45.4.411

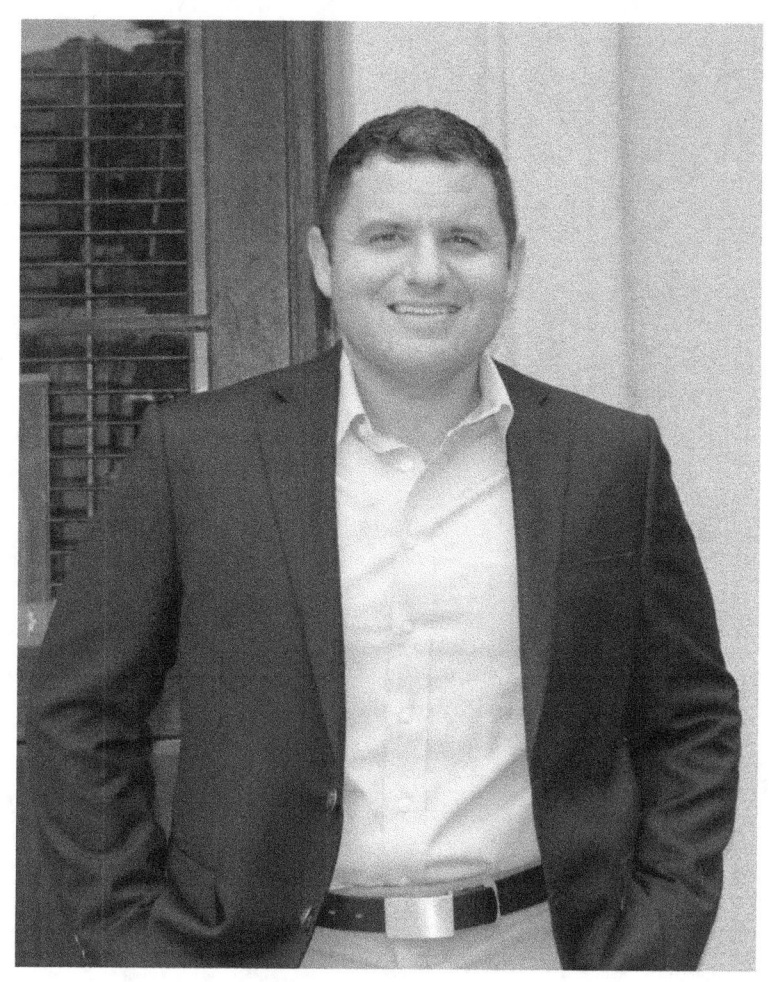

About the Author

This is the second book in *The Orange Book* series, the first being *The Orange Book of Louisiana Notary Exam Practice Questions*. Chad earned his Bachelor of Science degree in Athletic Training at Southeastern Louisiana University in 2007. He earned his Master of Arts degree in Health Studies at Southeastern Louisiana University in 2012. Chad served as an Athletic Trainer for Southeastern Louisiana University's football and baseball team between 2007-2008. He then served as Athletic Trainer at Brother Martin High School and the New Orleans Jesters of the National Premier Soccer League between 2008-2010. After earning his Master's degree in 2012, he taught in the Kinesiology and Health Studies department at Southeastern Louisiana University from 2012-2022. Between 2013-2022 he served as the Clinical Education Coordinator for the University's Athletic Training Education Program.

Chad Dufrene is the owner and operator of CAD Notary Services, LLC in Madisonville, Louisiana. He has performed mobile and remote online notary services in Louisiana since his commissioning in 2023. In 2023 he also gained an NSA Loan Signing Agent certification. Chad resides in Madisonville, Louisiana with his wife, Alyssa, son, Adam, and dog, Max. He can be reached at *cdufatc@yahoo.com*.